IDIOMS O

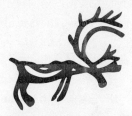

IDIOMS OF SÁMI HEALTH AND HEALING

BARBARA HELEN MILLER, *Editor*
EARLE WAUGH, *Series Editor*

Patterns of Northern Traditional Healing Volume 2

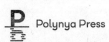 Polynya Press

An imprint of The University of Alberta Press

Published by
The University of Alberta Press
Ring House 2
Edmonton, Alberta, Canada T6G 2E1
www.uap.ualberta.ca

Library and Archives Canada Cataloguing in Publication

Idioms of Sámi health and healing / Barbara Helen Miller, editor;
Earl Waugh, series editor.

(Patterns of Northern traditional healing series ; volume 2)
Includes bibliographical references and index.
Issued in print and electronic formats.
ISBN 978-1-77212-088-2 (paperback). —ISBN 978-1-77212-104-9 (pdf). —
ISBN 978-1-77212-105-6 (epub). —ISBN 978-1-77212-106-3 (mobi)

1. Sami (European people) —Medicine--Europe, Northern. 2. Sami
(European people) —Health and hygiene—Europe, Northern. 3. Healing—
Europe, Northern. I. Miller, Barbara Helen, 1949-, editor II. Series:
Patterns of Northern traditional healing series ; v. 2

DL442.L3I35 2015   305.894'5745   C2015-905809-0
                                            C2015-905810-4

ISSN 1927-9671

Index available in print and PDF editions.

First edition, first printing, 2015.
Printed and bound in Canada by Friesens, Altona, Manitoba.
Copyediting and proofreading by Angela Wingfield.
Map by Wendy Johnson.
Indexing by Stephen Ullstrom.

The University of Alberta Press gratefully acknowledges the support received for its publishing program
from the Government of Canada, The Canada Council for the Arts and the Government of Alberta through
the Alberta Media Fund.

This work is published with the assistance of the Centre for Health and Culture, Department of Family
Medicine at the University of Alberta, as well as a grant from the Western Canadiana Publications Project.

 Government of Canada / Gouvernement du Canada

 Canada Council for the Arts / Conseil des Arts du Canada

Alberta Government

Generous funding assistance for this volume was provided by Ms. Marion Waller in memory of her beloved companion, Mr. Robert Aitchison.

Contents

Foreword

The circumpolar north today is a region built of stark contrasts. While it is often characterized by its climate, or even its harshness, each northern community demonstrates an attention to well-being, or even intimacy, which is thought to be absent in southern urban spaces. Set within one of the last great global frontiers of resource extraction, the circumpolar Arctic is awash in money and infrastructure, and yet northern communities are often the poorest or most vulnerable among northern nation-states. With this cacophony of contrasts it is sometimes hard to hear the local initiatives and ideas which lend resilience to northern lives. In this volume, Barbara Helen Miller has carefully drawn our attention to the plurality of approaches to healing—the idioms—that one can find in several Sámi communities. She presents a strong argument that communities subjected to colonization are never completely colonized. They harbour often unexpected approaches which lend a sense of balance and autonomy. The key to understanding these pathways, as every author here demonstrates, is through attending to and listening to the experiences—and dreams—of the local residents. The role of the inspirational Sámi "reader" is often to draw attention to the clues to which the patient is attuned. The role of this volume similarly is to direct our attention to avenues of healing which may be unexpected.

For those familiar with the literature on the circumpolar north, one of the more unexpected lessons in learning about Sámi healing strategies is the significant absence of drums, shamans, and medicine. This is an absence built of expectation and not attention. As Stein Mathisen outlines in his subtle cultural history of the colonial contact zone, northern Scandinavia for a long time has been an arena in which one hopes to find the survivals of lost traditions. This expectation itself disempowers local community actors, who, like everyone else, engage with the evocative traditions that work for them. Unlike in eastern Siberia or the Canadian Arctic, the power of texts and Christian rituals play an important role in northern Scandinavian communities. This is sometimes understood to be the result of acculturation—or of loss. This volume demonstrates that these qualities are instead a strength and a testament to the creativity of local healers.

The contributors to this volume, while cautious of institutional biomedicine, also recognize its value in certain circumstances. The healers Kjell Birkely Andersen, Sigvald Persen, and Barbara Helen Miller speak from their own experience to help their patients identify stories that explain their sense of fortune, as well as shed light on the social welfare ministries which provide the financial spaces for survival. Sámi healing in this idiom is not an autochonous, radical exercise which turns its back on the world, but it suggests a thoughtful appropriation of the available resources including some of those offered by a state that once brought colonization. This untidy picture of central institutions which sometimes colonize and sometimes offer respite is a common trope across the North, and one which requires more examples and more discussion to be understood fully. This series is a strong step in that direction.

The contributions to this book were assembled through a similarly untidy dialogue. The papers are based on a set of presentations made possible in part by an International Symposium grant from the University of Tromsø. A symposium, in June 2010, brought together students of the healing practices in three different regions of the North: eastern Siberia, Northern

Norway, and western Canada (through the thoughtful comments of the series editor, Earle Waugh). From our discussions and travel together then, I think we all remember our surprise at the very different ways in which difficult topics such as the use of alcohol, or the public attribution of landscape spirits, were handled in regions which many of us expected to be roughly similar. The symposium was held in an institution with a strong northern mandate. It has since been renamed the Artic University of Norway, yet it is probably not a secret that the large hospital and associated medical school based at the university is one of the stricter examples of a centralized approach to the delivery of services. This site, at once centralized and at the same time open and hospitable, was the site where two volumes of the Patterns of Northern Traditional Heading series were born. It is my sincere hope that this productive paradox will continue to inspire debate and attention to the idioms of health and well-being across the North. This volume is a sincere and powerful contribution to that end.

DAVID G. ANDERSON
University of Aberdeen

Preface

We are proud to bring you *Idioms of Sámi Health and Healing*, the second volume of the Patterns of Northern Traditional Healing series. This series is focused on addressing important health traditions of northern populations.

Readers have found the series helpful because it addresses a critical arena of knowledge that has been largely ignored in medical studies today. Although traditional Chinese medicine, for example, continues to attract widespread scholarly interest, local northern conceptions have been addressed by only a few dedicated specialists. While this state of affairs may be understandable given the scattered and fragmentary work done on circumpolar communities, there are striking reasons for remedying the situation.

The first is the increasing significance of development to northern communities. As global warming spreads northwards, small communities will feel the impact of a completely different and perhaps foreign culture. Resource exploration and development treats the landscape in ways that are not recognized by these traditional cultures. For many traditional peoples the landscape has therapeutic significance. Incoming cultural shifts could be socially disruptive and destructive. The more we know of the traditional ways before this impact dominates, the better we can assist the cultural change.

The second is the negative health outcomes in existing northern communities. Some of the most glaringly negative statistics in the world are found in these northern communities. It is evident that while allopathic medicine has had an impressive effect on many large populations, the medical picture is much more complicated. The perception is that older and established patterns of health are rooted in cultural needs and aspirations that embrace different meanings of well-being. The time may have come to join with these older and sustaining views in order to nourish and adapt so that health outcomes can be improved.

The third is the continued nurturing of health by these traditions in communities even though they are not "official." Many of the traditions have potency outside of government programs, and some have considerable loyalty among followers. Properly harnessed, they provide an untapped reservoir of knowledge with which to improve life expectancy and health outcomes. Moreover, the principles of compliance are built in; followers adhere to them because they are rooted in a long cultural history or are validated by local rituals.

Fourth, since they are often "below the radar," the traditions have a life of their own and obviously interact among local people in various ways, being validated by local folk and local authorities. They have striking resilience and have proven that they can survive even when official health organizations decry or publicly undermine them. And they appeal to a wide range of ages and personalities. A good example of the continuity of these traditions can be found among the indigenous people examined in this volume, the Sámi of northern Scandinavia.

These and other reasons motivate us to explore this rich layer of cultural meaning and bring it to a wider readership. We hope you find *Idioms of Sámi Health and Healing* to be insightful and engaging.

This volume is the second of five proposed studies of circumpolar regions. We continue to explore north Central Asian cultures and what they might tell us about the deeper layers of health strategies. An upcoming conference will address northwestern North America, bringing scholars and practitioners together in Edmonton, Alberta, to examine traditions from Alaska, the Northwest Territories, northern British Columbia, northern Alberta, and the Yukon. Our final conference will focus on northeastern Canada and Greenland.

EARLE WAUGH, Series Editor
University of Alberta

Acknowledgements

The editors would like to acknowledge the contribution of Dr. David G. Anderson, then of the Department of Anthropology at the University of Tromsø, for his kind willingness to host the conference on Sámi traditions that provided most of the articles published here. We are also grateful to the Faculty of Humanities, Social Sciences, and Education for the use of its facilities and for the International Symposium grant which made this first meeting possible; and to Marit Myrvoll and the Norwegian Institute for Cultural Heritage Research for their hospitality. We would also like to recognize the support of the Centre for Health and Culture, Department of Family Medicine at the University of Alberta for their sponsorship of the Patterns of Northern Traditional Healing series.

Without the assistance of Elaine Maloney, formerly of the Canadian Circumpolar Institute, this project would not have come to fruition. Lastly, the editors and authors wish to thank Angela Wingfield for making their text sing, and the University of Alberta Press, which continues University of Alberta's vital role in northern and circumpolar publishing with Polynya Press.

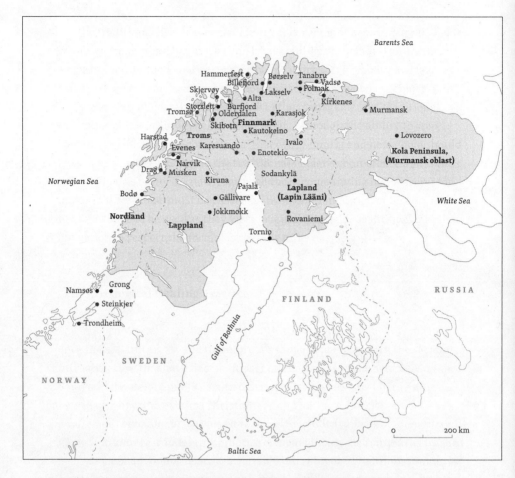

The shaded area shows Sápmi, the historical territory of the Sámi.

Introduction

BARBARA HELEN MILLER

The present volume is the second in the Patterns of Northern Traditional Healing series, following the book of essays entitled *The Healing Landscapes of Central and Southeastern Siberia*, which was edited by David G. Anderson and includes a preface to the series by Earle Waugh. Our essays reflect the work of a committed group of scholars who agreed on the value of providing a forum for discussing local idioms of health. Northern Scandinavian governmental research agendas have focused on epidemiology and considered how the health care in rural communities differs from that in urban settings, but they have not considered the strengths of the local communities' own resources for health and prevention. The authors hope to redress that lacuna.

The Sámi are the indigenous people of northernmost Europe, a people who have been dispersed and culturally divided. The Sámi language stems from the Uralic family, which contains two main groups, the Samoyedic languages and the Finno-Ugric language; the Sámi belongs to the latter. Several clear dialects exist within Sámi, of such diversity that it may be more accurate to speak of the Sámi group of languages. The geographical areas in which the present-day Sámi people live include the most northern provinces of Norway, Sweden, Finland, and Russia. Our essays report from the area of the highest concentration of the Sámi population, the Norwegian provinces of Finnmark, Nordland, and Troms; additionally, and experienced as fortunate, is one report from Kola, Russia, where the Sámi presence is greatly diminished and whence there has been no prior work published on the Russian Sámi approach to healing today. The diversity of the Sámi is such that the health investigation presented in each chapter of this volume is best read with application to the specified region. Future health studies are therefore all the more welcome so that other regions with Sámi populations may receive the attention that is their due.

Sámi culture has often been associated with reindeer herding, but, in line with the emphasis on diversity, the Sámi in the coastal regions have predominantly been fishing. Additionally, it was only after the sixteenth century when the stocks of wild reindeer became reduced that more Sámi specialized in herding to a greater extent; their nomadic practice had been documented as ongoing in previous decades (Hansen & Olsen, 2004). Many Sámi communities historically practised a semi-nomadic lifestyle, moving together between the mountain areas and the coastal areas according to the season. Other groups practised reindeer herding in forested areas. It was not uncommon to combine reindeer herding with hunting, fishing, and farming. Other Sámi combined fishing with small-scale farming (see Hætta, 1996, p. 20). So, in addition to specific local categories, the Sámi speak of Reindeer Herding Sámi and Coastal or Sea Sámi. In Norway the Sámi were Christianized predominately during the early-eighteenth century. In this period Norwegian settlements increased in the traditional Sámi areas, and today the Sámi are a minority group within Norway, Sweden, Finland, and Russia, where they number approximately 70,000 and are engaged in a variety of modern occupations.

Shamanism was an ingredient of the pre-Christian Sámi culture and of the pre-Christian "old" religion, which had a pronounced animal ceremonialism (in particular to the bear). The religion included sacrifices to the life-giving powers in rituals at special locations called *sieidi* in Sámi. There were sacred locations marked by dramatic natural formations, such as a rock or a steep canyon. Sámi religion would have been woven into everyday

social conduct, in which certain codes of respect toward *sieidi* were important. The pre-Christian Sámi term for the Sámi healer is (among others)
noaidi, and scholars conclude that the pre-Christian occupations of the
noaidi agree with the diverse social roles that can be assigned to the shaman
(Bäckman & Hultkrantz, 1978). While there are many similarities, there are
also differences between the shamanism of the Sámi and the shamanism
of other regions. For example, the Sámi shaman differed from the Siberian
shaman in not having any special attire. Also the initiation period did not
contain the experience of dying and dismemberment, and the *noaidi* did not
use the central world tree or pillar as a channel of communication with, or
of transportation to, the beyond. The Sámi shaman did employ the drum and
did enlist spirit helpers (see Hultkrantz, 1992). The category of shamanism
does not exist in a unitary form, and current scholars speak of a plurality of
"shamanisms" (Atkinson, 1992). A minimal definition of *to shamanize* can be
"to come into contact with the world of the gods and spirits through certain
preparations" (Bäckman & Hultkrantz, 1978, p. 69), but what is important
is that "shamanisms" are embedded in particular world views as well as in
wider systems of thought and practice.

Today the Sámi traditional healer most often considers himself or herself as Christian (drums were confiscated and forbidden predominantly
during the seventeenth century in Sweden and the eighteenth century in
Norway), and the healer is not referred to locally by the term *noaidi* or the
cross-cultural term *shaman* but by terms that translate as "improver," "one
who returns," "one who knows," and "reader." However, the Sámi healer is
still an inspirational healer. That there should be an uncomplicated line from
the former shamanic practice to the present-day healing tradition, though,
is untenable. Christianity also carries a legacy of inspiration. Amongst the
Sámi in some locations and areas the Christian line of change and continuity
in the practice of inspiration can be posited by the ongoing influence of
pietism. Pietism, a religious movement of the late-seventeenth and early-
eighteenth century in Germany, emphasized the need for a revitalized evan-
gelical Christianity and stressed informal devotional meetings (conventicles
called *collegia pietatis*), Bible study, and personal experience of God's presence
(see Brown, 1996). The Christian ethos that was influential in converting the
Sámi was that of pietism. Thomas von Westen (1682–1727) lead the mission to
the Sámi from 1716 to 1727 (Steen, 1954, pp. 422–432). Von Westen, the single

most important missionary to the Sámi, was influenced by pietism. A pietist revival movement from the Torne River Valley in Sweden reached Northern Norway during the 1770s (see Zorgdrager, 1989, pp. 107–108, and Outakoski, 1987, pp. 208–210). Lars Levi Laestadius (1800–1861), a Lutheran minister in northern Sweden, laid the foundation of a religious movement within the Lutheran Church. Laestadianism has been called the religion of the Sámi,[1] and its pietist roots are visible in the conventicles that encourage lay participation (emotional and enthusiastic); in conversion as a main tenet; and, perhaps most vitally, in the doctrine of the priesthood of all believers.

The complexity of viewing continuity in the world view of traditional Sámi healing includes not only an alternative to shamanism by the inclusion and influence of pietism but also the processes of acculturation within Laestadianism and traditional healing. The essays do not set out to establish syncretism[2] but do propose, by their focus on idioms and present-day practice, that there is a similar pattern of ideas and shared terminology within Laestadianism and traditional Sámi healing. In the present essays Marit Myrvoll marks the shared terminology of *gifts of grace*, and Miller of *baptism*.

The majority of the chapters in this volume view the Sámi traditional healer as an inspirational healer. In Chapter 2, Anne Karen Hætta shows that the Sámi traditional healer has charismatic authority; the villagers recognize the healer as qualified in terms of charisma. She explores the local understanding of the codes that indicate the esoterism of Sámi traditional healing, accompanied by special challenges for the transmission of that healing knowledge today. Considered by Hætta as possible precipitating elements in the present norm of secrecy are the earlier efforts to Christianize the Sámi, as well as the more recent Norwegian laws against the quacksalver.

Sámi healing strategies include the application of herbs and animal products, but our essayists have found the more prevalent activity to be that of what I am calling *inspirational healing*. However, any healer may use a combination of remedies that include plant and animal products. What may be unexpected to the etic view is the distinct lack of embrace by residents of Northern Norway of new shamanism (the reinvention or revival of shamanism that has some popular support in Europe). Myrvoll found in her area of research that traditional healers are without doubt Christians. In Chapter 4 she examines the understanding of these Northern Norwegian villagers of the transmission and management of healing knowledge, as demonstrated by "inheritance" and by Christian "gifts of grace." Additionally she clarifies the relatively new phenomenon whereby an individual professes to be a shaman, and lays out distinctions. Someone claiming to be a new shaman is viewed by locals as not connecting to Sámi tradition but as importing a non-Sámi tradition and/or working with evil spirits.

Another theme approached by the majority of the essays is the aftermath of colonization, in which there is a continuing lack of alliance between local traditions and biomedicine. In his contribution (Chapter 1) Stein Mathisen aims to understand how Sámi folk medicine was first established as a field of scholarly research. Healing knowledge was traditionally related through narratives; scholarly documentation of Sámi healing practices excerpted elements from the narratives, often in taxonomic order, creating a divide between magical and empirical medicine.

There are local conceptualizations for the presumed aetiology and the preferred treatment of ailments that do not follow the biomedical model of the division between mental health, bodily symptoms, and general well-being. Such local conceptualizations would be the aetiology of "ongoing bad luck" in which the causes identified varied from supernatural to natural to psychosocial. We can consider ongoing bad luck as a local syndrome; help is not sought within the biomedical health-care system for such conditions, which are expected to improve through support from traditional healers. Kjell Birkely Andersen, Sigvald Persen, and Barbara Helen Miller (Chapter 5) explore the uses of local healers and of psychiatry in Finnmark, showing changes and indications of resilience. The aetiology for experiencing a momentary paralysis is explored in Chapter 4, in which I show the dynamics of the practice that a healer has called "naming."

Chapter 6 by Trine Kvitberg, on the experience of health in the Kola Peninsula, employs the narrative of an elderly Kola Sámi woman. She experienced the displacement of her community and a rupture with the traditional reindeer-herding lifestyle. The narrative centres on the subsequent change in food consumption and relates this to health.

Changes in the social fabric of local life are particularly notable after World War II. Each geographical area has its own variations. In Porsanger Municipality prior to the war, Laestadian meetings, large and small, had been a central focus of social life; after the war, political parties (for example, the Labour Party) and sport associations, among others, were the more active arrangers of social life. Changes in the social life were particularly affected by the new welfare system introduced by the government, with regulations for all businesses. Prior to World War II the Sámi co-operative organization whose members worked and lived together, called a *siida*, had controlled a common resource territory that was used jointly for seasonal migration and for various resource niches (see Vorren & Manker, 1962). Presently only Reindeer Herding Sámi still bide by the *siida*. Also still in practice, but greatly reduced to be almost non-existent, is the traditional relationship that was maintained between reindeer herders and the Coastal Sámi, called *verdde* in Sámi, which is a reciprocal relationship between nomad and sedentary people (see Eidheim, 1971).

The relationship of psychiatry and traditional assistance is another theme in these chapters; in Chapter 8 Randi Nymo shows the bridging between traditional practices and science-based practices that is actively achieved by dwellers in the rural districts of the northern Nordland and southern Troms counties. There is an innovative process, as a consequence of generations of encounters by these dwellers with modernity, whereby "framing" a situation is a step toward agency. In Chapter 7, Mona Anita Kiil analyzes her findings from interviews of, among others, patients of a psychiatric outpatient clinic in a northern Troms community. She concludes that an ongoing negotiation tactic is employed by these patients in their use of traditional medicine with its spiritual and care component and of the clinic with its pharmaceutical and psychotherapeutic component. Ambiguities concerning the Sámi identity play a role in the patient's construction of "home," which is achieved by selective discourse.

Chapter 9 by Britt Kramvig brings us into the moment of creating culture, and the healing quality that this has for the community. This creative moment traditionally uses the dream, which achieves a reconnection to the community, and can be seen as an entrance into Sámi epistemic practices.

Resilience and continuity are ongoing themes in this book, and the chapters uncover an important layer of the health traditions that remain a part of Sámi idioms of health and healing in this part of the world. The chapters suggest important legacies that propose novel ways of addressing health issues among Sámi communities today.

Notes

1. As the Laestadian movement spread in Northern Norway, it maintained a non-ethnic stance, being actively inclusive of Finnish, Norwegian, and Sámi peoples.
2. Methodology for questions of syncretism are well formulated by André Droogers (2004) with his advocacy for viewing shared and changing repertoire and mental scripts for behaviour, thought, or emotion: schema.

References

Atkinson, J.M. (1992). Shamanisms today. *Annual Review of Anthropology, 21*, 307-330.

Bäckman, L., & Huktkrantz, Å. (1978). *Studies in Lapp shamanism.* Stockholm: Almqvist & Wiksell.

Brown, D.W. (1996). *Understanding pietism.* Nappanee, IN: Evangel Publishing House.

Droogers, A. (2004). Syncretism, power, play. In A.M. Leopold & J.S. Jensen (Eds.), *Syncretism in religion: A reader* (pp. 217-236). London: Equinox.

Eidheim, H. (1971). *Aspects of the Lappish minority situation.* Tromsø, Norway: Universitetsforlaget.

Hætta, O.M. (1996). *The Sami, an indigenous people of the Artic.* Karasjok, Norway: Davvi Girji.

Hansen, L.I., & Olsen, B. (2004). *Samenes historie fram til 1750.* Oslo: Cappelen Akademiske Forlag.

Hultkrantz, Å. (1992). Aspects of Saami (Lapp) shamanism. In M. Hoppál & J. Pentikäinen (Eds.), *Northern religions and shamanism* (pp. 138-145). Helsinki: Regional Conference of the International Association of the History of Religions, Finnish Literature Society.

Outakoski, N. (1987). Cuorvvot. In T. Ahlbäck (Ed.), *Saami religion* (pp. 208-210). [Vol. 12]. Åbo, Finland: Donner Institute for Research in Religious and Cultural History.

Steen, A. (1954). *Samenes Kristning og Finnemisjonen til 1888.* [Vol. 2]. Oslo: Avhandlinger utgift av Egede Instituttet.

Vorren, Ø., & Manker, E. (1962). *Lapp life and customs.* London: Oxford University Press.

Zorgdrager, N. (1989). *De Strijd der Rechtvaardigen: Kautokeino 1852.* Utrecht: Proefschrift University Utrecht.

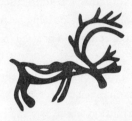

Constituting Scholarly Versions of a "Sámi Folk Medicine"
Research Practices in the Colonial Contact Zone

STEIN R. MATHISEN

The academic communities' understanding of Sámi indigenous healing practices has changed and transformed, as indicated by shifts in scholarly research initiatives. These shifts will be revealed through a historical retrospective, and it is important to note that the early documentation and representation of these practices have been coloured by research projects and theoretical understandings (be they written, exhibited, or performed). This chapter will take a closer look at how various actors, whether documenting or communicating, have worked to create cultural images, performances, and especially texts with the aim of communicating information related to this field of study. My view is that more attention should be paid to investigate the initiation of such projects and the kind of scholarly understanding that motivated them. This implies understanding the specific contexts and strategies that produced these representations and texts, and noting that the ideas emanating from documentation of Sámi folk medicine have in due course appeared in various other and new contexts, ultimately changing and transforming the original practices and turning them into something else. This is to say that the Sámi healing practices taking place in their Sámi local context will never be identical to their representation in a book, an exhibition, or a performance. In that sense the transmission and subsequent transformation of healing knowledge is an example of a colonizing activity, in which Sámi healing practices were taken out of context to be used for a new purpose and in a new context.

However, it is important to note that these extractions and documentations took place as a communication and an exchange between two parties, Sámi and non-Sámi. Even though the distribution of power was very uneven, and clearly one must speak of a hegemonic relationship, there was also agency among the colonized and suppressed indigenous populations. It is therefore important to understand some of the informants' actions as strategic and intentional. When indigenous specialists chose to share (or not share) their knowledge of Sámi healing practices, they had contemplated the consequences of such actions, calculating that the strategies for collaboration would not always be successful and that the conflicts could be insurmountable. This is a field of interaction and communication that should not be ignored, as it potentially holds ominous consequences also for future work in the border zone between indigenous and scientific medicine. A historical view of the cultural meeting places—where people from two different cultural backgrounds with very different access to power worked to produce versions of indigenous healing practices to be presented within the frame of Western science—holds teaching potential for any future enterprise within this field of documentation and research.

Transforming Indigenous Knowledge

In the eighteenth-century descriptions of Sámi healing practices, such activities were both condemned and valorized in a variety of ways. The scholar's attitude to the northern areas and their indigenous populations was often prejudiced and biased, and this has continued to leave traces to the present day. The attitudes seem to have rested on dual understandings of the Sámi, which were often ambiguous. On the one hand, a number of Christian descriptions condemned the Sámi for their heathen religion and understood their healing practices, in this religious confusion, as something superstitious or utterly primitive and pre-Christian (Schefferus, 1673/1956). From this point of view it was important to eradicate the "false" indigenous beliefs and substitute them with the "right" belief, namely the Christian faith. On the other hand, however, some descriptions from the eighteenth century praised the Sámi as a nature people and saw them as living in total pre-lapsarian and innocent harmony with nature. Thus the indigenous inhabitants of the European north were described as having specialized knowledge about using elements from nature, such as the plants and animal products available in their Arctic environment (Linné, 1732/1811). This was even seen as something that could be useful to the natural sciences, which were beginning to be established at that time.

The same kind of equivocal descriptions can be found in later writings about Sámi health conditions during the 1920s and the 1930s, sometimes referring to the healthy life of the nomadic Reindeer Herding Sámi (Qvigstad, 1932, p. 1), while at the same time portraying life among the more sedentary, Coastal Sámi as utterly unhealthy or inevitably causing illness and degeneration (Qvigstad, op. cit.). This is very much in accord with similar descriptions of indigenous populations and colonized peoples all over the world at that time and apparently parallels the understanding of indigenous people as representing "noble savages" on the one hand and "ignoble savages" on the other (see Ellingson, 2001).

What all these views had in common was that they were seen from the perspective of outsiders. From the outside, observers described Sámi everyday life experiences and tried to understand them within the frame of reference that they brought with them from their own religion, scientific knowledge, or general view of the world. These perspectives were also typically colonizing, in the sense that they sought to change the religious mindset of the colonized, to control the natural and mineral resources of the explored areas, or to benefit from people's indigenous knowledge so that they could be extracted and used for other purposes.

It was not an obvious fact that Sámi healing practices would constitute the separate field of study that was later labelled "Sámi folk medicine." Rather, this must be understood as a result of research practices, documentation strategies, archiving procedures, and other kinds of transformative actions in a cultural communicative field. In short, any of these operations meant dislocating the specific, localized practices related to indigenous healing activities. They were taken out of context, where they had been used as a part of everyday practice, and then re-established in new surroundings, for new purposes. Generally, this transformation is what Richard Bauman and Charles Briggs, with reference to folklore texts, identify as the processes of decontextualization and recontextualization (Briggs & Bauman, 1992). These processes imply questioning the attainment and use of power and authority that is used to change the previously established connections between context, actions, words, and meanings: "Producers of discourse assert (tacitly or explicitly) that they possess the authority needed to decontextualize discourse that bears these historical and social connections and to recontextualize it in the current discursive setting" (Briggs & Bauman, 1992, p. 148).

The research practices connected to Sámi healing customs should then be understood in a colonizing perspective, in which indigenous knowledge, like any other resource, is being exploited for the production of new surplus values in completely new surroundings.

This transformation and dislocation of knowledge could sometimes be violent and forceful, as in the missionaries' burning of the *noaidi's*[1] drum and the desecration of Sámi holy places. However, it could also occur in the form of peaceful transactions, even if the power was very unevenly distributed in this relation. When it comes down to real encounters between living beings, the meeting between the colonizer and the colonized must also be understood as a type of communication. From both sides certain strategies were being applied to convey their message, so to speak. For this reason the literary theorist Mary Louise Pratt chose to substitute the term *colonial frontier* with the concept *contact zone*, to "foreground the interactive, improvisational dimensions of colonial encounters so easily ignored or suppressed by diffusionist accounts of conquest and domination" (1992, p. 7). A central point here is that the informants as well as the collectors used certain strategies that motivated them to continue their communication, even if it was taking place "within radically asymmetrical relations of power" (op. cit.). This raises questions such as what is being communicated in which context, and for what purpose. But it also raises the question of what the limitations might be to these kinds of cultural encounters.

The present analysis aims primarily to understand something of the context in which Sámi folk medicine was established as a field of scholarly research, with a special focus on identifying the various strategies applied by the actors from both sides in meetings that took place in the colonial "contact zone." The material has been chosen from a selection of texts dealing with indigenous Sámi folk medicine in different periods, but in one way or another they can all be seen as the result of a kind of colonial meeting between the representatives of a majority population and an indigenous people. In addition, they can all be identified as contexts in which the collection of indigenous healing practices produced texts that became formative for the later understanding of what the field of Sámi folk medicine would find to be relevant and would include.

Systema Naturae
Linnaean Understandings of a Nature People and Their Knowledge

The knowledge of Sámi healing practices emerged as a field of study that was built upon contributions from various fields. A substantial amount of the knowledge on earlier shamanistic and magical healing practices among the Sámi that has accumulated in literature and archives today originates from the writings of precisely those people who worked most actively to eradicate these beliefs. This can be seen, for example, in the protocols from the witch hunts that took place in the seventeenth century (Rutberg, 1918), and in the reports made by missionaries and clergymen on various "heathen" religious activities (for an overview of this material see Rydving, 1993). Many of these activities were related to healing, but they were subsequently interpreted as typical examples of heathen worship or as contact with devilish powers, resulting in the firmly established image of the Sámi sorcerer within the European world view (Moyne, 1981).

However, some of the early descriptions by missionaries and clergymen pointed to other aspects of Sámi healing, which seemed to have little to do with their "heathen activities." An example of this can be found in the writings of the Swede Johan F. Körningk from Prague, who was involved with the Catholic mission (Körningk, 1660/1918, pp. 155–158). He writes that the Sámi are very able doctors and relates a narrative about a young man who was completely paralyzed until the age of eighteen. Then he was miraculously healed:

Ein Lappenartzt stellte ihn durch Anwendung gewisser, bei uns wenig geschätzen Kräuter so völlig her, dass er es fürder mit jedem im Laufen und Springen aufnahm. Dass ist nur ein Beispiel ihrer Wunderkuren. Ich habe mehrere dieser Heilmittel mit nach Prag gebracht. (Körningk, 1660/1918; here cited from Qvigstad, 1932, p. 24)

A Lapp doctor healed him completely with the use of certain herbs, not valued much among us, so that he afterwards could catch up with anyone in running and jumping. That is only one example of their wonder cures. I have brought with me many of these healing remedies to Prague. (Author's translation)

Further, it turned out that Körningk himself had been miraculously healed by his Sámi doctor. Suffering from a seriously swollen foot due to frost injuries, he received help for his ailment, which was so effective that the swelling disappeared completely overnight. Whereupon the Sámi healer had assured him that without this remedy he would surely have died (op. cit.). What is significant here is that "many of these healing remedies" could be brought back to Prague, clearly with the intention of putting them to use in new contexts and also of making the remedies work within a new frame of religious understanding. How was this transformation from a primitive and heathen context to a civilized and Christian context made possible?

With the early nature scientists a new way of understanding the surrounding world, its nature, and its peoples emerged. These scientists were open to the possibility that the Sámi as a nature people could hold some empirical knowledge that eventually would prove beneficial to professional medical practice in the future. It must be remembered that scientific medicine was still in its infancy. One such early nature scientist was the famous botanist and physician Carl von Linné (1707–1778). His great interest in the "nature medicine" of the Sámi is evident in the diaries of his first travel through parts of the Sámi area in 1732 (Linné, 1732/1811). Reading this diary, however, also reveals that Linné is in the process of actively constructing a certain narrative, set in more mythical surroundings, in which the Sámi take on the role of nature people and in that capacity become the proponents of a new narrative, invented and set in motion by Linné himself. This narrative holds both the new Linnaean understanding of nature as a system and the elements of a new economic understanding of the North and its indigenous population. He thought that these areas for Sweden could serve the same purpose as the overseas colonies did for the other prominent powers in Europe, and supply the country with the necessary resources and goods for its further expansion (Koerner, 1999). Linné further saw the Sámi combination of life in nature, their diet, and their medicine as an ideal and proposed that in many cases the Sámi could act as models for people who had become too used to life in the cities and had been "destroyed" by civilization and the consumption of foreign goods. Linné is supposed to have maintained that "the Lapps are our teachers" (Koerner, 1999, p. 76), and this is the rhetorical version of the myth of the Noble Savage that was actively chronicled by Carl von Linné himself. By applying some of their medical remedies, and not least by describing his own medical practice as a version of Sámi indigenous healing, he not only "focused on the economics of colonization" but also started the "appropriation of indigenous medicine" (Koerner, 1999, p. 63).

During his travels in Europe in 1735–1738 Carl von Linné publicized himself with great success as a physician who had mastered an unknown medicine originating from a nature people, the Sámi (Koerner, 1999, p. 56). It is also significant that on the frontispiece of his book *Flora Lapponica* (Linné, 1737), he is pictured in the middle of a Sámi landscape, dressed in what appears to be Sámi dress, and holding the *noaidi* drum on his lap. A similar motif can be found in a 1737 portrait, which Linné commissioned from the Holland painter Martin Hoffman; he is fully dressed in his Sámi costume and has the *noaidi*'s drum attached to his belt. Judging from the available sources, Linné usually wore this costume during his stay in Holland; it was assembled from various "souvenirs" of Lapland that he had obtained many years after his "Iter Lapponicum" (Koerner, 1999, p. 66). The obvious constructed nature of this dress parallels his construction of a narrative of the fruitful combination of indigenous knowledge and his own discovery of a system of nature. More important, however, it was an ingredient of Linné's personal performative narrative that he used to introduce himself to the learned society in Europe as someone coming from the periphery of Scandinavia. At the same time, it is the image of the colonizer masquerading as the colonized (Koerner, 1999, p. 64) and purporting a narrative of anti-conquest (Pratt, 1992). Carl von Linné created an image of a scientist who was deeply influenced by Sámi indigenous healing practices and who also had a colonizing view on how the area and its resources could be used to the sole benefit of the Swedish nation.

These general ideas of finding valuable knowledge about nature from a nature people inspired further investigations from science and medicine. In 1734 Johannes Fjellström of Sweden presented his dissertation *Medicina Lapponum* at the University of Lund based on investigations in Pite- and Ume-Lappmark, and in 1751 a pupil of Carl von Linné, Lars Montin (1723–1785), defended his historical-medical dissertation *Medicina Lapponum Lulensium* and earned a doctoral degree, also at the University of Lund. Montin observed that every nation or ethnic group had some medical remedies that were peculiar to that group or region, and he maintained that scientific attention to this might lead to important discoveries, even if the ethnic group holding this knowledge was in its most barbarous state (Montin, 1751/1758, p. 733). He further concluded that the Sámi whom he investigated seemed to be totally ignorant of anatomy and physiology but to have a wide knowledge of remedies (taken from both plants and animals) that could be used for the healing of their illnesses. The use of magical cures does not, however, seem to fall under the category of what Montin wants to term *medicine*.

This divide between magical and empirical medicine runs through much of what has been written later about Sámi healing practices, even as the authors often have difficulty in maintaining the logic of such dualistic taxonomies. When the healing practices are analyzed in relationship to the narratives and understood in their cultural contexts, they often turn out to be combinations of "rational" and "spiritual" ways of understanding illnesses. It was important for scientific medicine to sort out this indigenous "misunderstanding" in order to establish the rational and medical elements that, after all, could form the basis of a medicine that could be found useful in despite of its primitive origin.

The Lappologists and a New Scholarly Colonization of Sámi Healing Practices

In his time, the Norwegian folklorist and philologist Just Knud Qvigstad (1853–1957) was considered to be one of the most prominent and respected collectors of Sámi folklore. His name has been associated with a group of scholars called the Lappologists as *Lapp* at that time was the dominating international, scholarly term for the Sámi ethnic group. The Lappologists were usually occupied with extensive empirical documentation within the fields of language, culture, ethnography, and (physical) anthropology. While *Lappology* in its time was considered to be the neutral and unbiased term describing this field of research, the contemporary use of the term often bears with it connotations of cultural colonialism, owing to Social Darwinist attitudes, extensive collections of Sámi skeletal remains, large projects on comparative physical anthropology in anatomical institutions, and so on. All of these activities point to the present-day realization that much of this work is best understood through the perspective that Lappology was not unbiased but was part of the efforts to colonize the Sámi areas in terms of resources as well as culture.

Qvigstad was born in a small fjord community in Northern Norway called Lyngseidet, on the Lyngen fjord in the northern part of Troms County. It was then a multi-ethnic and multilingual community, consisting of people with Sámi, Kven (Finnish), and Norwegian backgrounds. The young Qvigstad was in a privileged position because he was the son of the district physician who had moved to the area for professional reasons, and at the age of 21 he graduated in Old Norse, Greek, Latin, Philosophy, History, and History of Literature from the University of Kristiania. He secured a teaching position at Tromsø Seminarium (later known as Tromsø Teachers' College), with a special obligation to teach the Sámi language. Qvigstad later became headmaster of the college, a position he held for several decades (Nesheim, 1971). In his work he adhered to the idea that a schoolteacher who was proficient in the Sámi language would be better equipped and therefore instrumental in improving the level of schooling in Norwegian in the traditionally Sámi-speaking areas. Many of the most gifted Sámi students accordingly received scholarships to be trained as teachers and were eventually placed in teaching positions in the areas from which they had originated. If the intention was to contribute to what in Norway is termed the "Norwegianization" of the Sámi population, in many cases this was probably a successful strategy.

From another perspective, however, it is interesting to see how these Sámi teacher students also became cultural intermediaries and played various and sometimes more contradictory roles in the colonizing process. In addition, some of the Sámi students became great resources for their local Sámi communities and contributed politically and culturally to a strong revitalization and strengthening of the Sámi culture and language. One example of such a prominent former student is Anders Larsen (1870–1949), who was a schoolteacher in three different Sámi areas of Northern Norway; he is also known as the author of the first novel in the Sámi language (Larsen, 1912) and as the editor of the Sámi newspaper *Sagai Muittalægje*, which was established to counter the effects of Norwegianization. Another prominent student of Qvigstad was Isak Saba (1875–1921), a schoolteacher from Nesseby who in 1906 became the first Sámi representative in the Norwegian parliament. Both of these former students became important assistants to Qvigstad as folklore collectors. While Qvigstad himself had collected some of the Sámi folklore material in the field, these prominent former students collected most of the material for him according to questionnaires he had created, and helped him to document it (Qvigstad, 1896). This often gave the collected material a certain structure or order that corresponded to the themes and questions already set up by Qvigstad in the questionnaires. The inherent "logic" of these questions was based not so much on local, contextualized Sámi thinking or world view but rather on the scholarly theories that reigned in the folklore studies and ethnography at that time. These decontextualizations of Sámi folklore material can be seen, however, in a double perspective when it comes to their printed recontextualizations.

Qvigstad's collection of Sámi folk medicine is one of the results of this extensive documentation of Sámi folklore, and its organization is typical of the way in which the Lappologists would make use of the narrative material that they gathered. The collection is based on excerpts from all available written sources that mentioned the subject, as well as on collections made by Qvigstad himself and by his data-collecting former students and on material that he had obtained from his fellow Lappologists in the Nordic countries. Not only did the method take the narrative texts out of their context (decontextualized), a context in which they had communicated a specific meaning, but also the narratives were "chopped up" and presented under new headings or subjects. Qvigstad, after a rather short introduction on shamanistic and magical healing methods among the Sámi (Qvigstad, 1932, pp. 6–23), presents the rest of the book, more than two hundred pages, divided into sections devoted to different medical diagnoses. Under these headings are presented short descriptions of ailments and cures from all over the Sámi area.

This recontextualization eventually created completely new meanings. Unlike the contexts in which the Sámi folk medicine had been collected, the book's presentation of "magic" medicine was clearly divided from that of the medicine using plants or parts of animals. This was again represented as either an irrational or a rational cure, according to the current status in scientific biomedicine at that time.

The joint folklore-collecting project between Qvigstad and his former students resulted, as mentioned, in an impressive collection, and most of it was published in Qvigstad's name (for an overview of some of this production see Mathisen, 2000a). Still it seems paradoxical today that Qvigstad often expressed negative views concerning the status of this folklore treasure. Despite having devoted a long lifespan to collecting and publishing numerous volumes on Sámi folklore, he was convinced that Sámi culture and language would perish within a short time. He further maintained that most of this material was not genuine Sámi but had been borrowed from the Sámi's neighbouring peoples (Mathisen, 2000b, p. 188). In conclusion he writes as follows about the background of the Sámi healing practices that he has documented:

> *Wenn man die Volksmedizin der Nachbarvölker der Lappen betrachtet, kann die Antwort nicht zweifelhaft sein: die Hauptmasse ist entlehnt. Wie in Betreff des Aberglaubens und der heidnischen Religion, der Sprache und der Kultur sind die Lappen die Lehrjungen und ihre Nachbaren die Lehrmeister.* (Qvigstad, 1932, p. 227)

When the folk medicine of the neighbouring people of the Lapps is examined, one can have no doubt about the answer: most of it [Sámi folk medicine] is borrowed. As with their superstitions and their heathen religion, their language and their culture, the Lapps are the pupils, and their neighbours are the teachers. (Author's translation)

It is important to note that folklore studies as a subject had been established in Norway to support the idea of a national culture. The first

professor of folklore in Norway, Moltke Moe (1859–1913), was the son of
one of the first two famous folklore collectors in Norway, Jørgen Moe
(1813–1882), who together with Peter Christen Asbjørnsen (1812–1885) published the first collections of Norwegian folklore; thereby they both paved
the way for developing Norwegian national sentiments and inspired the
work of advancing a Norwegian written language. Molkte Moe became
an important person also in the ideological work of building the "new"
Norwegian nation-state. When Qvigstad, together with the clergyman
Georg Sandberg (1842–1891), published the first collection of Sámi folk
tales and legends in Norwegian (Qvigstad & Sandberg, 1887), Professor
Moe, as the absolute scholarly authority on the subject at that time, wrote
the preface, in which he maintained the following:

> Således har også lappefolket modtaget en overmåde stærk tilførsel
> af eventyr fra et folkefærd, som er det overlegne i kultur og
> kulturforbindelser; thi i regelen er det det mest fremskredne folk,
> som er det givende, og det mindre udviklede, som er det modtagende.
> (Moe, 1887, p. x)

> In this way the Lappish people have received a very heavy supply
> of folk tales from groups of people who are superior to them in
> culture and cultural contacts. Because the rule is that it is the most
> advanced people who are the donors, and the lesser developed who
> are the receivers. (Author's translation)

In relation to the collecting efforts made by Carl von Linné 150 years
earlier, the roles in the mythical classroom with the Sámi and their neighbours now seem to have been reversed. The Sámi had been positioned as
teachers and authorities on aspects related to their own culture by Carl
von Linné and the early nature scientists, but, with a new narrative turn,
the scholarly representatives of a modern, Norwegian national culture had
now turned the Sámi into subordinate pupils of a neighbouring people who,
for more than a century, had additionally managed to take more and more
control over their lands and resources.

The German scholar and Scandinavianist Norman Balk (1894–1975)
managed to have his book on Sámi folk medicine (*Die Medizin der Lappen*,

1934) published only two years after the appearance of Qvigstad's book. He acknowledged the scholarly authority of Qvigstad that had made his own work superfluous. All the same, he chose to publish it because he disagreed with Qvigstad on the point that most Sámi folk medicine had been borrowed from the neighbouring peoples *to the south*. Balk maintained that their oldest healing methods, for example shamanistic rituals and rituals involving moxibustion, should point toward their possible "Mongolian" origin. In that sense Balk's organization of the information on Sámi healing practices is in accord with another prevailing cultural theory at the time, that the Sámi had immigrated from the east. This theory also effectively placed the Sámi somewhere outside the land in which they now lived and worked, opening up and legitimizing the colonization of Sámi areas for other groups of people.

A similar kind of collecting and classifying endeavour can be seen in the work of Ludwig Kohl-Larsen (1884–1969). A German physician, he spent a year in Tana (Deatnu) in Finnmark, Norway, in 1925, working as a district physician, and subsequently reported his observations of "Sámi medical art" in the area where he had worked (Kohl, 1926a and 1926b). His work is filled with the contradictory sentiments that follow from an ambiguous position in relation to the field because he acted as both a teacher of modern principles of medical treatment and as a documenter of traditional healing methods. When he later had attained a position as a renowned ethnographer (Renner, 1991), he returned to Finnmark as a part of the occupying German military forces in 1943, with the title "scholar in military service" (Renner, 1994, p. 277). He amassed large collections of Sámi folklore during this stay (see further on this in Mathisen, 2000b, 198ff.). However, the very extraordinary context of their establishment implied that this communication faced problems in its transformation into conventionalized textual folklore products. The communication was eventually framed as that of an outside ethnographer who had observed the local culture, listened to narratives, and then categorized according to the existing rules of the scholarly community. Kohl-Larsen, himself a part of the occupying forces that left Finnmark with everything having been destroyed and burned, found that his documentation had a hard time being used as a basis for an intercultural communication and dialogue.

Sámi Folk Healing as Anti-colonial Strategy

From the pioneering work of Johan Turi (1854–1936) and onwards, one can more clearly observe the dilemmas of rendering a traditional, localized, and often esoteric knowledge in the media of writing and printing. Most interesting in this connection are Johan Turi's two books, *Muittalus samid birra*, which was first published in 1910 in an edition with parallel Sámi and Danish texts, and *Lappish Texts*, which was first published in 1918–1919 in an edition with parallel Sámi and English texts. Both books have large sections on the subject of Sámi folk medicine. They are generally understood to be the first written descriptions of Sámi culture made by a person who was a Sámi and who was also known to practise folk medicine. It is interesting in this context to note that Turi shows knowledge of the complex, transcultural reality of which Sámi healing activities had already become a part, as well as an awareness of the complex relations in which these healing activities would become involved if they were to be transported (or recontextualized) into other contexts.

Some of Turi's reflexivity may have arisen from the circumstances that produced the books. The books are actually the result of a very interesting co-operation between three persons. The Estonian folklorist Kristin Kuutma has written thoroughly about this co-operation in her book *Collaborative Representations* (2006), so in this context I will only focus on what is related to the question of healing practices. Johan Turi might have dreamed for a long time about writing a book to make the life of the Sámi known to the people who had colonized the Sámi areas. He wanted to turn people's attention to the values represented in Sámi life and culture. However, he was not able to realize this dream until he met the Danish artist and hobby ethnographer Emilie Demant-Hatt (1873–1958) in 1904. She had taken a great interest in the life of the Reindeer Herding Sámi and wanted to study their way of life. She became a whole-hearted supporter of Turi's idea of writing the book, and she also edited the notebooks that he had put together. The third party in this venture was, surprisingly enough, Hjalmar Lundbohm (1855–1926), director of the LKAB iron mining company. Although the company was perhaps the biggest colonizer in those Swedish Sámi territories, Lundbohm was still a strong supporter of the old Sámi reindeer-herding culture and very enthusiastic about Turi's book project. He furnished Turi and Demant-Hatt with a cabin to be used as writing quarters, and financed the printing of the book.

In this way the process of making the first book about Sámi life, written in the Sámi language by a Sámi, really can be understood as an enterprise taking place in what Mary Louise Pratt has called "the contact zone" (1992, p. 6), referring to the space in which colonial encounters are occurring. This is not to hide the fact that both domination and conquest are part of the colonizing efforts, but rather our point is to pay attention to the communicative strategies that the colonized have been able to use in this situation. Pratt also uses the term *autoethnography* "to refer to instances in which colonized subjects undertake to represent themselves in ways that engage with the colonizer's own terms" (1992, p. 7).

Some of the tensions that must have been part of the complicated creative process of Turi's book, and indeed the whole process of co-operation with the representatives of the colonizers of his land, even if they were positive to his project, are visible in the way that certain themes were presented by Johan Turi in the first book. This is especially true when it comes to the healing practices that constitute an important part of the presentation of Sámi culture and life. Before he starts presenting some of his healing knowledge, Turi reflects upon the way in which it is going to be understood by the learned community to whom he presumably is directing his words:

> *Men det lämpar sig inte att skriva upp alla konsterna i denna bok, därför att denna bok kommer at läsas över hela världen, och många lärda herrar passa inte att höra om alla konster, de tro inte på dem, bara håna lappens dumhet, fast om de finge se allt, vad lappen gör, så skulle de förundra sig över den kraften och varifrån den kommer.* (Turi, 1917, p. 115)

But it would not be appropriate to write about all arts in this book, because this book is going to be read all over the world, and many learned masters are not fit to hear about all arts; they would not believe in them, only mock the stupidity of the Sámi. But if they were able to experience everything a Sámi is capable of doing, then they would wonder about the force and where it comes from. (Author's translation)

Later in the text Turi explains that in this book he has described all the Sámi's healing arts but not their *noaidi* arts (p. 129). He explains that when the usual methods of healing were not effective, people believed that the illness had been caused by evil people sending dead people to torment them. These kinds of illnesses required the use of *noaidi* arts. Turi goes on to relate narratives of people who had sought the help of a *noaidi*, one of whom was the well-known Johan Kaaven who was active in Porsanger on the Norwegian side of the border (Turi, 1917, 133ff.).

Some years after the publication of the first book Johan Turi, again with Emilie Demant-Hatt, was planning the second book. As it turned out, the above-mentioned examples of narratives on *noaidi* arts were also elements that entered the book through Demant-Hatt's editing. Turi's reluctance to publish the more secretive and esoteric part of his folk medical knowledge is also referred to by Demant-Hatt in her preface to the second book:

> A large part of the present material has been in my possession since 1908 when I collected the material for JOHAN TURI's "Muittalus Samid Birra". This is the case with most of what belongs to "noaide-art" and "medicine." I could not publish this at the time, because JOHAN TURI had handed over to me his noaide-knowledge as a gift which I personally might use, but with the injunction not to publish it, because then it would "lose its power." I took only a few pieces, of a less secret nature, from this private manuscript and edited them in M.S.B. [*Muittalus samid birra*], this book supplementing the present collection in certain peculiars. (Demant-Hatt, 1919, p. 3)

This corresponds to a more detailed description of the relationship between the ethnographer and her informant, turning it more into a relationship between a sage and his disciple. Concerning the process of making Johan Turi's book, Emilie Demant-Hatt later wrote:

> *Jeg nevnte før, at Turi var troldkyndig, og om disse hemmelige Ting fortalte han mig meget—han gav mig af sin Viden som en Gave, da han mente, at jeg havde "stærkt Blod," og hvis vi slog os sammen, kunde vi blive et "dygtigt Noaidde-Par, som kunde helbrede Mennesker."*

Men de Ting han fortalte mig om de skjulte "Kunster" maatte ikke offentliggøres, "saa mistede de deres Kraft." (Demant-Hatt, 1942, p. 107)

I mentioned earlier that Turi was well versed in witchcraft, and he told me much about these secretive matters. He gave me of his wisdom as a gift, as he thought I had "strong blood," and if we were to combine forces, we would become a very "gifted pair of noaidis, able to heal people."

But the things he told me about the hidden "arts" should not be made public, because then "they would lose their powers." (Author's translation)

The second book was called *Lappish Texts* (Turi, 1919). It was "a collection of raw material" (Demant-Hatt, 1919, p. 4), which was planned to be directed more toward the scholarly establishment and thus become material for the research society. This was the group of "learned masters" of whom Turi (in his own words, *"opam hærat"*) had been sceptical in the preparation of the first book but who then turned out to be the most positive audience of the book. Together with Demant-Hatt, he seemed to have changed his views about the kinds of materials that it would be wise to include in the book. Emilie Demant-Hatt writes about this in the preface to *Lappish Texts*:

Nine years have passed, however, since JOHAN TURI presented me with his noaide-knowledge, and these many years have not failed to leave their mark on JOHAN TURI. Although he has not quite understood what it means to be a successful author, still his ambition has been stimulated by many persons encouraging him continually to follow up his luck as an author. In M.S.B. he has certainly disburdened his mind of what he had most at heart, and therefore he has not been able to act on the encouragements; but his ambition has been tickled. And then I asked him now for his permission to publish the "noaide-knowledge," there was no hindrance. (Demant-Hatt, 1919, p. 3)

Johan Turi seems to have had the idea that some sort of collaboration would be possible with the Danish ethnographer, not only concerning the

writing of the book but also within the other field that was of great importance to him—healing people of their illnesses. With the publication of the
first book, however, this project had changed slightly. Now it turned into a
project of publishing all the secret knowledge of the *noaidi* arts that Johan
Turi knew. Traditionally, it would not have been possible to make this
knowledge public without risking the loss of healing powers, but, according to Emilie Demant-Hatt, Turi now saw himself as having entered a new
status, that of a writer: "his ambition had been stimulated by many persons
encouraging him continually to follow up his luck as an author" (Demant-
Hatt, 1919, p. 3). It is possible that Turi had hopes of bringing the relation
with the Danish ethnographer to a whole new level, which would eventually
not only heal individuals but be a healing factor in the relation between the
Sámi and their Others, or between the colonized and their colonizers. As
some of the most important factors in the folk medical treatment of illnesses
are concerned with the healing and balancing of relations—between people
and supernatural beings, between the living and the dead, or between
people themselves (Mathisen, 2000c)—it is not surprising that the author
and healer Johan Turi saw his books as a possibility for healing some of
the severe consequences of the colonial projects that he and his people had
been experiencing. In that sense one can see his literary project as an act of
autoethnography, a term used by Mary Louse Pratt "to refer to instances in
which colonized subjects undertake to represent themselves in ways that
engage with the colonizer's own terms" (Pratt, 1992, p. 7). Turi's books are
typically dialogical in the sense that they try to create a larger understanding of the Sámi life and culture among the colonizing majority populations.
At the same time he wants his own people to remember the elements of
knowledge that could be in danger of vanishing.

Representing Sámi Healing Knowledge in a Post-Colonial Perspective

These attempts to take a closer look into certain historical endeavours in
order to document and describe the healing practices of the Sámi demonstrate that the outcomes must be understood as the result of the very
specific circumstances that produced them. The documenting contexts

were most often those characterized by the colonizing relationship and the uneven distribution of political power. At the same time, however, the field of Sámi healing practices offers a very interesting area of investigation for improving the understanding of the nature of the cultural colonization of the Sámi area. The power to define the epistemological status of the collected material was common in the scholarly community. This might lead us to view the historical material in a different light and to question its value as a source of knowledge of indigenous healing. Nevertheless, by contextualizing the material in new ways, we may also provide the present scholarly community with new knowledge and even raise some new questions concerning the role of healing practices in the colonizing process.

The contextualizing anew of former collections of Sámi folklore has already been proposed as a method by folklorist Coppélie Cocq, who has worked to "re-voice" the Sámi narrators of the past (Cocq, 2008). It is possible to reinstate these Sámi informants into the discourses in which they actually participated at the moment of initial documentation. This might be a hypothetical venture, reaching for a goal that might not always be possible to achieve down to every detail, but some of the power structures involved in the intercultural meeting of a dominated and minority Sámi culture and a dominating scholarly society can be reconstructed, as the examples above have shown. To look at the old archived and printed material on indigenous Sámi healing practices from a new angle might contextualize this material in relation to alternative understandings of the status of these collections.

The folklorist Thomas A. DuBois has written an interesting analysis (2010) of the texts on Sámi healing practices that were contained in Johan Turi and Per Turi's *Lappish Texts* (Turi, 1919). The study of texts, healing procedures, and narratives certainly reveals that many of these can be traced back to foreign (especially Scandinavian and Finnish) influences, particularly when it comes to the incantations (DuBois, 2010, p. 18ff; see also Mathisen, 2007, p. 8). However, DuBois interprets these "borrowings" from a perspective that is quite the opposite of Qvigstad's (1932). Far from Qvigstad's colonizing perspective on Sámi folklore texts as only borrowings from their culturally superior Scandinavian neighbours, he suggests that "an examination of the images of healing in *Sámi deavsttat* [*Lappish Texts*] illustrates the multicultural, historically inflected, and interculturally contested world that Johan Turi lived in, one in which he struggled to maintain and defend a distinctive Sámi identity even while meeting with and adopting many cultural features from surrounding and encroaching populations" (DuBois, 2010, p. 13).

This places both the texts about healing and the healing practices as products of the contact zone (Pratt, 1992). They were the meeting grounds where many different groups of people—as a result of migration (voluntarily or forced as a result of the establishment of new national borders) or the colonizing efforts of hunting for the rich natural resources of the area—were at each other's mercy. In that sense, there are similarities between the healing practice of reading incantations to treat illnesses, and the production of literature (ethnography or folklore) as a way of treating the negative consequences of colonialism in the Sámi area. This understanding places the narratives as well as the printed texts in the middle of the specific contexts that produced them, and not only as memories of a past culture that represented primitive thinking.

We emphasis the texts about healing practices as products of the contact zone because the procedures that we have witnessed in much of the early documentation of Sámi healing practices differ in nature. The procedure exhibited most frequently included extracting elements from indigenous knowledge, identifying them as belonging to old and primitive thinking, categorizing them in a new order, and then introducing them in a contemporary scientific structure. The scholarly documentation of Sámi healing practices excerpted elements from the narratives, often in a taxonomic order, so that illnesses and treatments could be listed in a manner that would satisfy the needs of a scientifically oriented research community, whether it was in medicine, ethnography, or folklore. These processes of decontextualization and recontextualization were not simply processes of translation or transformation; they were also processes of change that involved, and were deeply connected to, issues of power relations, colonialism, and forced dislocations. The products emerged as something else, and "Sámi folk medicine" turned out to be something epistemologically different from the Sámi healing practices that supposedly were their origin.

What is needed is to put these collected elements from Sámi healing practices back into the narratives of which they were once a part, and to understand these narratives in relation to the dynamic and changing circumstances that produced them. Healing knowledge was traditionally shared through narratives, in which illnesses and other misfortunes could be related to a wide range of contexts, to relations between people and ethnicities, and to different natural and environmental conditions (Mathisen, 2000c). In the perspective of post-colonial theory, these narratives must be interpreted in relation to the colonizing efforts that brought important cultural changes, with their challenges, to the areas in which the indigenous population lived. As it turns out, narratives relating to healing practices might be an important communicative field to improve the understanding of the contexts that once produced those practices.

Note

1. For the Sámi term *noaidi* the cross-cultural term *shaman* has been scholarly employed by, among others, Bäckman and Hultkrantz (1978). Employing the term *shaman* for *noaidi* is certainly problematic (see Miller, 2007). However, when keeping in mind a minimum definition (*to shamanize* was "to come into contact with the world of gods and spirits through certain preparations" [Bäckman & Hultkrantz, 1978, p. 69]), the convention is acceptable, even if it might be misleading in understanding present-day local discourse.

References

Bäckman, L., & Hultkrantz, Å. (1978). *Studies in Lapp shamanism*. Stockholm: Almqvist & Wiksell.

Balk, N. (1934). *Die Medizin der Lappen* (Arbeiten der deutsch—nordischen Gesellschaft für Geschichte der Medizin, der Zahnheilkunde und der Naturwissenschaften 11, herausgeben von Prof. Dr. med. et phil et med. dent. Fritz Lejeune, Köln). Greifswald, Germany: Universitätsverlag Ratsbuchhandlung L. Bamberg.

Briggs, C.L., & Bauman, R. (1992). Genre, intertextuality, and social power. *Journal of Linguistic Anthropology, 2*(2), 131–172.

Cocq, C. (2008). *Revoicing Sámi narratives: North Sámi storytelling at the turn of the 20th century* (Sámi Dutkan 5). Umeå, Sweden: Umeå University.

Demant-Hatt, E. (1919). Preface. In J. Turi & P. Turi (1918-1919), *Lappish texts* (pp. 3-4). Copenhagen: Bianco Lunos Bogtrykkeri.

Demant-Hatt, E. (1942). Johan Turi og hvordan Bogen "Muittalus Samid Birra" blev til. *Fataburen, 194*, 97-108.

DuBois, T.A. (2010). Varieties of medical treatment and hierarchies of resort in Johan Turi's *Sámi deavsttat. Journal of Northern Studies, 1*(2010), 9-43. Umeå: Umeå University, The Royal Skyttean Society.

Ellingson, T. (2001). *The myth of the noble savage*. Berkeley: University of California Press.

Fjellström, J. (1734/1758). *Tentatio academica sistens medicinam Lapponum*. (Lund.) Printed in A. Hallerus (Ed.), *Disputationes ad morburum historiam et curationem facientes VI* (pp. 711-730). Lausanne 1758.

Koerner, L. (1999). *Linnaeus: Nature and nation*. Cambridge, MA: Harvard University Press.

Kohl, L. (1926a). Ärztliche Kunst bei den Lappen. In L. Kohl, *Nordlicht und Mitternachtsonne: Erlebnisse und Wanderungen in Lappland* (pp. 125-140). Stuttgart: Verlag von Strecker und Schröder.

Kohl, L. (1926b). Heilmethoden und Aberglauben bei den norwegischen Lappen. *Münchener Medizinische Wochenschrift, 4*(Juni 1926), 957-959. Munich.

Körningk, J.F. (1660/1918). Ein Missionsversuch in Lappland. *Die Katholischen Missionen*, nr. 4-7. Freiburg.

Kuutma, K. (2006). *Collaborative representations: Interpreting the creation of a Sami ethnography and a Seto epic* (FF Communications 289). Helsinki: Suomalainen Tiedeakatemia.

Larsen, A. (1912). *Bæivve-Alggo: Muittalus*. Kristiania (Oslo): Grøndahl.

Linné, C. von. (1732/1811). *Lachesis Lapponica or a tour in Lapland*. London: White & Cochrane.

Linné, C. von. (1737). *Flora Lapponica*. Amsterdam: Salomon Schouten.

Mathisen, S.R. (2000a). Changing narratives about Sami folklore: A review of research on Sami folklore in the Norwegian area. In J. Pentikäinen et al. (Eds.), *Sami Folkloristics* (NNF Publications 6) (pp. 103-130). Turku, Finland: NNF.

Mathisen, S.R. (2000b). Travels and narratives: Itinerant constructions of a homogeneous Sami heritage. In P. Anttonen, A.-L. Siikala, S.R. Mathisen, & L. Magnusson (Eds.), *Folklore, heritage politics, and ethnic diversity: A Festschrift for Barbro Klein* (pp. 179-205). Botkyrka, Sweden: Multicultural Centre.

Mathisen, S.R. (2000c). Folkemedisin i Nord-Norge: Kulturelt fellesskap og etniske skiller. In I. Altern & G.T. Minde (Eds.), *Samisk folkemedisin i dagens Norge: Rapport fra seminar i regi av Institutt for sosiologi og Senter for samiske studier, Tromsø, 26-27 Nov. 1998* (Sámi dutkamiid guovddás / Senter for samiske studier skriftserie nr. 9) (pp. 15-33). Tromsø, Norway: Universitetet i Tromsø.

Mathisen, S.R. (2007). Folklore in northern multicultural contexts. *FF Network, 32*, 3-9. Helsinki: Folklore Fellows, Finnish Academy of Science and Letters.

Miller, B. (2007): *Connecting and correcting: A case study of Sami healers in Porsanger*. Leiden, Netherlands: CNWS.

Moe, M. (1887). Indledning. In J.K. Qvigstad & G. Sandberg, *Lappiske eventyr og folkesagn* (pp. iii–xxix). Kristiania (Oslo): Alb. Cammermeyer.

Montin, L. (1751/1758). *Dissertatio historico-medica de medicina Lapponum Lulensium* (Lund). In A. Hallerus (Ed.), *Disputationes ad morburum historiam et curationem facientes VI* (pp. 731–744). Lausanne 1758.

Moyne, E.J. (1981). *Raising the wind: The legend of Lapland and Finland wizards in literature.* Newark: University of Delaware Press.

Nesheim, A. (1971). J.K. Qvigstad (1853–1957). In D. Strömbäck (Ed.), *Leading folklorists of the north* (pp. 323–338). Oslo: Universitetsforlaget.

Pratt, M.L. (1992). *Imperial eyes: Travel writing and transculturation.* London: Routledge.

Qvigstad, J.K. (1896). *Veiledning til Undersøgelse af Lappernes Forhold.* Kristiania (Oslo): Grøndahl.

Qvigstad, J.K. (1932). *Lappische Heilkunde* (Instituttet for sammenlignende kulturforskning, Serie B, Skrifter XX). Oslo: Aschehoug.

Qvigstad, J.K., & Sandberg, G. (1887). *Lappiske eventyr og folkesagn.* Kristiania (Oslo): Alb. Cammermeyer.

Renner, E. (1991). *Ludwig Kohl-Larsen, der Mann der Lucy's Ahnen fand.* Landau, Germany: Pfälzische Verlagsanstalt.

Renner, E. (1994). Nachvort. In L. Kohl-Larsen, *Das Leben des Rentierlappen Siri Matti—von ihm selbst erzählt* (pp. 273–283). Aufgezeichnet von Ludwig Kohl-Larsen. Herausgeben von Erich Renner. Frankfurt and New York: Campus Verlag.

Rutberg, H. (1918). Häxprocesser i norska Finnmarken 1620–1692. *Bidrag till kännedom om de svenska landsmålen ock svenskt folkliv, 16*(4), 1–110. Stockholm: P.A. Norstedt & Söner.

Rydving, H. (1993). *Samisk religionshistorisk bibliografi.* Uppsala: Uppsala universitet.

Schefferus, J. (1673/1956). *Lappland.* Trans. Henrik Sundin. (Acta Lapponica VIII). Uppsala: Gebers / Almqvist & Wiksell.

Turi, J. (1910). *En Bog om Lappernes liv. Muittalus samid birra.* Stockholm: AB Nordiska Bokhandeln.

Turi, J. (1917). *Muittalus samid birra: En bok om samernas liv* (Lapparne och deras land VI). Uppsala: Wahlström & Widstrand.

Turi, J., & Turi, P. (1918–1919). *Lappish Texts.* Edited by E. Demant-Hatt. Copenhagen: Bianco Lunos Bogtrykkeri.

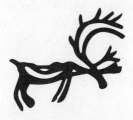

2

Secrecy in Sámi Traditional Healing

ANNE KAREN HÆTTA

I remember the summer after my father died. I was in his room in the old house, my niece and I. I was there and rummaged around, and in a closet I found a bunch of papers. There were a lot of love letters from my mother, and I started reading them. By chance I found his written healing instructions.[1] It was a pile of yellowed papers, and I started reading them. When I started reading, all the letters flew into one another, and it was just like someone was grabbing me around my neck and choking me. I thought, "Oh my God," and threw the papers away. I thought this is just nonsense; this is just something I am imagining. I tried to read them again, and the exact same thing happened. It was a sign that I should not touch it.

This story was told by the daughter of a traditional healer in the Marka villages, and her interpretation of the experience was that her father was still watching over his instructions and that she should stay away from the healing inscriptions because they were not intended for her. Years later, the story was well known within the family and was also referred to by the younger generation to illustrate that traditional healing knowledge is not intended for everyone. The story indicates that one should respect the secrecy of this knowledge and not try to gain insight into it when it has not been offered by the former owner.

Introduction

There is much focus on the preservation of traditional knowledge among the Sámi today, as more and more knowledge is forgotten and disappears with the changes to the livelihoods, technology, and everyday life of the people. Accordingly, much effort is put into the collection and documentation of traditional knowledge, with the intention of making it available for younger generations who have not had the chance to obtain it through the "traditional" way. A type of knowledge, however, that has not received much attention when it comes to safeguarding Sámi traditional knowledge is the knowledge that is held in secret or esoterically.

To explain the different characteristics of Sámi traditional knowledge Marit Myrvoll (2000, 2009) suggests three degrees of openness. The first, *available knowledge,* is generally open to everyone. The second, *withdrawn knowledge,* which is not regarded as common knowledge, is maintained in closed arenas to which few outsiders have access; this knowledge can be connected to the oral storytelling tradition and includes, for instance, dreams, visions, experiences, and stories about underground people and ghosts. Finally, *secret* or *esoteric knowledge* is something into which only a few chosen individuals are initiated, and the explanations and the reason for secrecy are often of a mythical or religious character. Part of what is held as secret knowledge in the Sámi culture is traditional healing knowledge, which is the focus of my study.

Owing to the secret nature of traditional healing knowledge, it is often not available or suitable for the same kinds of preservation and revitalization projects as are other types of traditional knowledge. It would, for instance, be difficult to have access to it for the purpose of documentation and dissemination. If the aim is to safeguard[2] traditional healing knowledge, I find it relevant to try to understand the reasons for such knowledge being kept secret. This chapter examines the secrecy norm in traditional healing and elaborates on some of the reasons for it.

The essay is based on my master's thesis (2010) about the management and transmission of traditional healing knowledge in specific Sámi communities in the Marka villages of southern Troms and northern Nordland, Norway. The geographical areas on which I have focused consist of several smaller villages in the outlying areas on the Stuornjárga peninsula and belong to the Skånland (Skánit, in Sámi) and Evenes (Evenášši, in Sámi) municipalities. The data was collected over four weeks in the period of August and September 2009, when I conducted semi-structured interviews with 15 individuals. Among them were three traditional healers and several other possessors of healing knowledge, in addition to others who had a close relationship to traditional healing and traditional healers.

Sámi Healers and Traditional Medicine

The World Health Organization (WHO) makes a division between traditional medicine and complementary and alternative medicine (CAM). It defines traditional medicine as "the sum total of the knowledge, skills, and practices based on the theories, beliefs and experiences indigenous to different cultures, whether explicable or not, used in the maintenance of health as well as in prevention, diagnosis, improvement or treatment of physical and mental illness" (WHO, 2005). CAM is described as "a broad set of health care practices that are not part of a country's own tradition and are not integrated into the dominant health care system" (ibid.). These definitions imply that what is considered to be traditional medicine in one culture would become alternative if exported to another country or culture. Chinese medicine, for example, is regarded as traditional in the country of its origin, but it becomes alternative in the Western countries.

Sámi traditional medicine cannot easily be differentiated from other traditional medicine in the same region, and many of the healing practices and techniques found among the Sámi are also found among other ethnic groups and in distant cultures. Traditional medicine in Northern Norway is formed by the Sámi, Kven, and Norwegian traditions, and Mathisen (2000) argues that the mutual influence they have had on each other stems from traditional medicine being an open system in which anyone can seek help regardless of their ethnicity and religious convictions.

Myrvoll (2000) has nevertheless made a distinction between three categories of Sámi healers that belong to different time periods and different religious contexts: the *noaidi*, the traditional healer, and the neo-shaman. In her opinion the old *noaidi*,[3] also called the Sámi shaman, does not exist any more in the form described in the old sources about Sámi pre-Christian religion; the *noaidi* tradition as a cultural phenomenon, however, has adapted to religious change. The modern-day traditional healer is working in a Christianized society, and Myrvoll argues that in the areas with which she is familiar the traditional healers have to choose to work for "God" or "the devil." She sees continuity in the selection of the present-day traditional healer and the old *noaidi*: both were appointed or selected by others, and the selected ones often showed resistance to their vocation.

Myrvoll further states that the Sámi neo-shamans are influenced by neo-religiosity, as they seek out and pick up ideas and elements from a range of different religions. They are, however, also incorporating content, values, and traditions from the pre-Christian Sámi religion, including rituals and ritual objects connected to it. She argues that even if the tasks of the *noaidi* and the neo-shaman could be seen as partly overlapping, there are crucial differences in the management of the tasks and of the knowledge. While the knowledge of the *noaidi* and the traditional healer is held in secret and is esoteric, many neo-shamans are conveying their knowledge openly through workshops and courses.

There are many different terms for the Sámi traditional healer, and the name varies between different areas and groups. Some of the terms used in Northern Norway are in the Norwegian language—*leser* (reader), *hjelper* (helper), *blåser* (blower)—and some are in the Sámi language—*guvhllár* and *buorideaddji* (one who makes better). I will here use the Sámi name *guvhllár* interchangeably with *traditional healer*. *Healer* is a term that has (locally and in the press) come to be associated with a healer operating in the field of CAM, and therefore I qualify my use of that name for those who practise CAM.

Methods and Traditions

The forms of treatment within Sámi medicine are varied and diverse, and traditional healers can use multiple techniques. It is told that there are *guvhllárs* of different degrees of power, and they could also specialize in different diseases or problems; for instance, they could be better at curing infections, blood poisoning, toothache, or pain. Not every facet of traditional medicine was conducted by a *guvhllár*; for example, herbs and plants were open for anyone to use for healing or preventative purposes. Materials that have been in use in Sámi traditional medicine include wool, ash, bone, urine, alcohol, tobacco, blood, feces, hair, and other parts of animals (Steen, 1961). Methods used among the Sámi could include *ruvven* (massage), *varra luoitin* (bloodletting), and *duovlut* (tinder burning).

The most common methods within traditional healing in the Marka villages today are *lohkan* (reading), the laying on of hands, and *vara bissehit* (blood stopping). A *guvhllár* who practises reading heals by reading prayers or formulas, most often quietly in order to keep them esoteric. These consultations are done in the home of the *guvhllár* or that of the afflicted, but the reading may also be done from a distance when the *guvhllár* is contacted by telephone or mail. Some *guvhllárs* are described as having "warm" or "electric" hands, and they can combine reading with the laying of their hands on the patient. Blood stopping is also practised by the reading of particular secret formulas and prayers, and earlier this process was quite common among the Sámi. A person who knows how to stop blood is not necessarily regarded as a *guvhllár*, and Mathisen (2000) aligns the knowledge of blood stopping to a less esoteric category than that of other traditional healing knowledge. As blood stopping can be life saving in emergencies, it was probably necessary that it was more widespread than other healing knowledge.

A *guvhllár* can also have knowledge beyond purely medical matters, and it is believed that some are able to help find lost things or persons, as well as to make thiefs immobile or make them bring back what they have stolen. A *guvhllár* can furthermore be contacted for "cleaning" houses when spirits are believed to be occupying them (Sexton & Buljo Stabbursvik, 2010). Many of the situations they deal with, however, can represent social and relational problems, which again are indirectly connected to physical and mental well-being.

While working as a psychologist in a Sámi community, Torild Hanem (1999) often found that mental illness was explained as someone having inflicted or placed *neavrrit* (Sámi for "evil") on another. It was not unusual for her patient to visit a *guvhllár* or another helper to handle the *neavrrit* both before and during the therapy with her. A related belief is that some people can affect others by the power of thought, and this phenomenon is widely known as *gand* in Norwegian and as *gannja* in the local Sámi dialect in the Marka villages. *Gannja* has been described as a potential tool for justice when the one on whom the *gannja* has been placed had broken some social norms in the community (Nergård, 2006). Both these beliefs have been seen as traces of the old Sámi religion and the *noaidi* tradition (Miller, 2007; Nergård, 2006).

The phenomenon of *gannja* is something that remains in the consciousness or world view of people in the Marka villages. I was told several stories of people having had *gannja* or evil put upon them, and that it explained the strange behaviour of animals and otherwise unexplainable incidents, accidents, or diseases. Even though most of the stories were from the "old days," *gannja* was mentioned also, by both older and younger people, as a possible explanation for currently occurring happenings.

The Transmission of Traditional Healing Knowledge

There are several ways in which a traditional healer would have received his or her healing abilities. Mathisen (2000, pp. 20–23) elaborates on two parallel explanations. First, the transmission can be seen as a vocation from the forces, that is, as one chosen by God. Conceptualized within the Christian language it is said that a person receives a "gift of grace." Other accounts imply that a *guvhllár* has been taught by "the underground people" or has received the gift by unidentified powers.

Second, there is an emphasis on the inheritance and transmission of healing abilities. It is believed that the qualities for becoming a *guvhllár* can be inherited in particular families or that the traditional healer will choose a successor. Inheritance also includes the passing down of knowledge that is held to be esoteric (ibid.). The transmission of this knowledge can include teaching by an older *guvhllár*, with or without the inheritance of written instructions of traditional healing methods. There can also be cases in which healing abilities are passed on and received via a dream after the death of the former *guvhllár*.

The general idea is that traditional healing knowledge cannot be taught to someone older than you and that there can be only one inheritor of the knowledge. However, an older female *guvhllár* whom I interviewed was of the opinion that it was possible to teach it to several persons but that the healing power would be distributed, becoming weaker each time. For that reason it was not desirable to teach it to too many people.

The Qualifications of a Rightful Successor

As some *guvhllárs* are believed to have knowledge by which they can harm others and themselves, it is underlined that this knowledge cannot be shared with just anyone. One of my young informants thought that young people were afraid of the knowledge because "it is said that those who can do the good things also know how to do the bad things. I would not have liked to learn, because I would have misused the knowledge if someone, for instance, insulted me." People in the Marka villages had their own understanding of what it takes to be a *guvhllár* candidate and a qualified inheritor of the healing knowledge. A trait that was often emphasized was that it had to be a "good" person. As one of the villagers stated, "one cannot be evil, because then you can put *gannja* on others. We had a woman here, before our time. She was evil, and she used to put *gannja* on everyone if she did not get it like she wanted."

Even though the villagers may have their opinions about it, the individual carrier of the knowledge is the one who makes the decision as to whom he or she will transmit the knowledge. The carrier has his own considerations about the kind of qualities that the successor should have, and who would be able to fill the role of a traditional healer and handle the knowledge adequately. An older male *guvhllár* explained: "You feel those in a crowd of children you can transmit it to." He holds that if they show interest in the knowledge, then they have it in them; this means that they have a spiritual side and want to help people. Another *guvhllár* with whom I spoke said that a candidate must really understand the implications of being a *guvhllár*; she also emphasized that it has to be someone who will maintain and use the knowledge, not just keep it passive. My understanding of her opinion is that showing general interest is not enough; the candidate must show a deeper understanding and be prepared to accept the role.

Having extraordinary capacities was a recurring response when I asked about the qualities that a traditional healer candidate should have, and these capacities could be manifested through sensitivity to supernatural phenomenon. One of the *guvhllárs* maintained that for cupping and reading one did not need to have special abilities, but it was an advantage if one saw and heard more than others did. She also considered that the knowledge should be assigned to a person who did not tell and reveal everything.

Traditional healing has been surrounded by secrecy and taboos, and the communication of the norms and values in this tradition has happened most often when people are discussing those whom they feel have crossed these lines. The criterion of secrecy informs the opinions about a suitable inheritor of the knowledge, as that one must be a reliable person with respect to both holding the knowledge esoteric and using the knowledge properly. There are, however, different kinds of secrecy and different levels of a secret. One part of the secrecy is connected to the possession of the healing knowledge or healing abilities. The degree of secrecy and the explanations for it can be very different from the degree of and explanations for the secrecy connected to the content of the knowledge.

Secrecy About Possessing the Knowledge

In my fieldwork I noted that the local *guvhllárs* were seldom known to everyone in the village and that people referred to different individuals when talking about the traditional healers whom they directly knew and used. Therefore, the "publicity" of the *guvhllár* varies, and while some are more or less official traditional healers in the villages, others are very private and are not known outside their family and closest friends.

A traditional healer should never say out loud that he or she practises healing, and, when contacted by a patient, a *guvhllár* would never answer, "Yes, I will help you," but rather something like, "I will try to do what I can." Most of my informants opined that they did not believe in those who talked, advertised, or bragged about their abilities. Some believed that it had something to do with not putting oneself in focus, because many traditional healers refer to themselves as helpers or as instruments of a greater power by which the healing is done. Some identify this force as God, while others refer to it as an unknown power. For that reason it is important to show humility for their healing abilities and their role as a traditional healer.

Many of the carriers of traditional healing knowledge prefer to keep a low profile for different reasons. Some are afraid that it can be a struggle to be a well-known *guvhllár*, as one *guvhllár* whom I interviewed found it to be. She said that she preferred to keep her abilities low key, explaining that treating people took a considerable amount of time and that the commitments of her family life and full-time job were taxing enough. Another *guvhllár* admitted that it became exhausting when people called, and not all healers wanted to spend their time and energy on this. They might feel they do not have the capacities for healing, or they could be worried about being in the public spotlight. This *guvhllár* also explained that there was a responsibility when one had special capacities, and there could be people who did not have enough self-confidence for the role. He said, "People have certain expectations of a *guvhllár*, and one needs to be able to withstand it."

The contraindication for speaking about their abilities also has roots in the history of the Sámi. When the missionary work and Christianization of the Sámi intensified in the late-seventeenth and early-eighteenth centuries, all practices and material expressions with connections to the Sámi religion were prohibited, being seen as "Sámi sorcery." As a result, rites and Sámi conceptions that could be associated with Sámi sorcery were forced into a tabooed context and then practised only very privately (Hansen & Olsen, 2004, p. 318). The death penalty for Sámi sorcery was abolished in Norway in 1726, but the Sámi were given fines and corporal punishment for using drums and for sacrificing. The missionaries aimed particularly at Christianizing the *noaidis* and in the process confiscated drums and sacred objects and destroyed sacrificial places. Conflicts among the Sámi also arose as some of them co-operated with the missionaries and reported those who continued their old religious practices (Rydving, 1995, pp. 54–68).

However, the prosecution of persons believed to have command of witch-craft and sorcery had started even earlier. The witch trials in Europe had spread to Northern Norway at the end of the sixteenth century, and during the period of 1593–1682, a total of 177 people were accused of sorcery in the three northernmost counties; 126 of these were sentenced to death. Finnmark County was overrepresented in the witch trials in Norway, something that has been explained by an idea about the centre of the evil being situated in the north, and the Sámi being particularly talented in sorcery (Blix Hagen, 2005; Hansen & Olsen, 2004, pp. 324–327). Although the majority of the accused were non-Sámi, Sámis were often mentioned during the trials. Strikingly, many of those accused in Finnmark claimed to have learned their skills from Sámi women, who often lived in the counties further south (Hansen & Olsen, 2004, p. 327).

The criminalization of Sámi traditional healing has continued to the present time. In Norway until 2004 there were restrictions in place that pro-hibited anyone other than doctors and dentists from treating health problems. The Medical Quackery Act (Kvaksalverloven) of 1936 was finally replaced in 2003 by a new law that included alternative treatment. This law still gives the public health sector the exclusive right to treat serious diseases and illnesses, but it accepts alternative treatment in addition and allows individuals to make a choice when seeking treatment for less serious illnesses (Act 64 of 27 June 2003 relating to the alternative treatment of disease, illness, etc.).

The colonial and assimilation history can also be relevant, especially in areas exposed to harsh Norwegianization. Using traditional medicine and having extraordinary capacities have been part of the ethnic categorization of Sámis in this area (Mathisen, 1983), and in that context there has been an ethnic stigma connected to practising traditional medicine and healing. One of the older *guvhllárs* in the Marka villages saw this connection between the politics of assimilation and the stigmatizing and shaming of certain practices; she remonstrated that it used to be treated as nearly sinful to make use of the Sámi healing tradition, and that people had been scared of admitting to its use. In addition, traditional medicine has been regarded as backwards and primitive, and such healers have felt rejected and nullified when they have spoken about their experiences, especially clairvoyance, for which they have been diagnosed as having a mental disease (Minde, 2000, p. 100).

Sanctions for Breaking Norms

The secrecy norm has been most clearly demonstrated by the way in which people speak about those who break the norm, who advertise and promulgate their healing abilities. The villagers seem to clearly differentiate the traditional healers in whom they "believe" from those who do not follow the local norms. These persons are called humbugs and quacks and are considered to be only interested in doing business. There are consequences for a *guvhllár* who does not follow the local norms and values; he loses respect among the group, and eventually people stop asking him for help. *Guvhllárs* can be sanctioned by the community by people questioning their motivations for practising their gift; or their healing abilities are denounced.

During my fieldwork I found that some of those who were believed to possess traditional healing knowledge were hesitant about speaking with me, but there were others who did not have misgivings about engaging in the project. There are many examples of *guvhllárs* having talked to both researchers and journalists about their healing practices, and an obvious question to ask then is, if the secrecy norm is really so important, why do some *guvhllárs* still agree to be interviewed?

In my assessment, among the traditional healers who agreed to talk to me to a certain degree were well-known *guvhllárs* who accordingly had solid recognition as traditional healers from the community. We could conjecture that people who are well established and respected as traditional healers might have more confidence in their role and be relatively more accustomed to talking about traditional healing outside their closest circle. They perhaps have more self-assurance in (or even knowledge about) determining how much they can say and in how much detail. That their role as traditional healers has already been legitimized by the community appears to be of importance when it comes to the amount of information that they share openly.

Snåsamannen[4] engaged the media about his healing practices, but this did not seem to influence the way in which the people of the Marka villages assessed his healing abilities. Some of my informants were of the opinion that because he had been practising as a traditional healer long before the media attention began, it was unlikely that he was actively trying to attract customers; rather, his interest lay in the spreading of information. Others reacted negatively as a result of this media attention. However, it still does not seem to have affected the credibility of Snåsamannen to a larger extent, and none of my informants really doubted that he had healing abilities. One of the *guvhllárs* was rather positive of the fact that Snåsamannen had been so open about it, because it encouraged others to speak freely about it also. He said, "Just as I now dare to talk to you."

I believe that an important factor in the continuing recognition of Snåsamannen among the Marka villagers is that his position had been legitimized by the time he entered the media spotlight, and his healing abilities were widely known and credibly demonstrated. He has also repeatedly claimed that he does not take payment for what he does, because he accordingly would lose his healing abilities (VG Nett, November 20, 2008). In this respect he has demonstrated that he holds the same values that are important to the Marka villagers. Perhaps for this reason he can take the liberty of saying more than do those who do not occupy such a solid position in the community and command such respect; his capacities and intentions have already been proven.

Secrecy About the Content of the Knowledge

In his analyses of the guru and the conjurer, Fredrik Barth (1994) presents two contradicting principles in the management of knowledge. The gurus, who are Muslim teachers in Bali, wish to share their knowledge with as many people as possible because in this way the knowledge will be strengthened. The aim is to inspire their audience by spreading the word, explaining, instructing, and being a good role model for their successors. The conjurer knowledge that Barth found among priests in New Guinea was enhanced when it was protected, and it was shared only by a few. The conjurers consequently keep their knowledge esoteric and only display it during short revelations in small, closed assemblies. Barth views the guru and the conjurer as social roles with completely different requirements for their fulfillment, roles that are culturally constructed from their respective belief systems.

The knowledge management of the traditional healers in the Marka villages is comparable to that of the conjurers; however, the reasons for holding the knowledge as esoteric can be diverse. The secrecy of the healing knowledge can be explained by different factors, and the explanations are, in particular, grounded in religion and the belief system. According to Sámi tradition, one of the reasons for holding traditional healing knowledge esoteric is that not everyone is strong enough to handle the knowledge, and there can be a "knowing too much." Another important reason for holding knowledge secret is the conviction that those who know how to do good things, as in healing, also have the knowledge and capacities to do bad things. Traditional healers are expected to use their knowledge to do good and, as a rule, to prevent the opposite. People with the wrong intentions should accordingly not gain access to it. The holders of knowledge have been instructed to keep the knowledge secret and have learned the rules of transmission. They have been taught that if secrecy is not respected, they can lose the ability to practise the gift, or their abilities will weaken.

Scholars are often inclined to analyze secrecy as being a means to gain power. Georg Simmel (1950, pp. 332–333) maintains that when some people are excluded from knowing, it creates a strong feeling of possession for the insiders; it also communicates to the outsiders that the secret is highly valuable. The ones who hold the secret are given an exceptional position, which enhances a socially determined fascination. The contents of the secret are not necessarily important, because the outsiders are not privy to such details, and the contents may, in fact, be fictitious or even non-existent.

The power that traditional healers might hold in the community is connected to both the respect and the fear of what they (or the forces with which they are in contact) have the ability to do. Clairvoyance can be seen as a source of anxiety, mainly because of people's speculation about what a person with this gift might know about them or others. Not knowing exactly the content of the *guvhllár's* knowledge reinforces this effect, as do stories about traditional healers and the narratives of personal experiences with a *guvhllár*.

It is then conjectured that the power of traditional healers would only have an effect on those who believe in traditional healing. Sociologist Max Weber (2005) differentiates between three types of social authority, by which he means the power to affect other people's actions by their will. They are traditional authority, rational-legal authority, and charismatic authority. The motivations that people have to obey the authority can be based on their conviction of the correctness of the instruction, on a feeling of obligation or fear, on habit, or on the desire for personal benefits. Weber argues that every social authority must receive justification by some right to rule. The position of the Sámi traditional healer in his terms would be justified and legitimized by charismatic authority. Charismatic authority is grounded in devotion to an individual person and his or her charisma, appearing as magical powers, revelations, heroism, the power of the spirits, or the power of the word. These extraordinary capacities are recognized on the basis of their demonstration in wonders, and the leader is only obeyed as long as he or she is acknowledged and ascribed these special qualities (ibid., pp. 98–104). When applied to Sámi traditional healing, if the *guvhllár* loses his charisma or fails to prove the power of the spirits, the authority is indeed lost.

Charismatic authority can also be transferred to a successor in that the carrier of charisma can designate someone. Other options include the choice of the successor by the disciples or followers, by a special method, or by heredity, in the belief that the charismatic capacities lie in the blood. What is important here is that the validity of the authority is legitimated by the fact that the followers recognize the individual person as qualified in terms of charisma. The authority of a traditional healer is only valid inside his or her group of followers and as long as the group recognizes the charisma as being real.

Maintenance and Protection of the Secret

According to Simmel (1950), the secret is always surrounded by the possibility and temptation of its being revealed, which will be the climax in the development of the secret. What he regards as most interesting, from a sociological aspect, is individuals' capacity or inclination to keep the secret to themselves, which is influenced by the relationship of preserving and yielding energies in a human relation. He argues that a feeling of superiority lies in the secret itself, and this feeling is only fully actualized in the moment of revelation.

When it comes to the knowledge of Sámi traditional healers, there does not seem to be the same kind of temptation connected to the revelation of the secret. Most people to whom I talked in the Marka villages seemed to respect the reasons given for the secrecy of the knowledge, and they also understood that reception of the knowledge was something that came with clear obligations and that it was not something to be taken lightly. The belief that one can lose the healing powers if speaking publicly about the knowledge is also important in keeping it concealed.

Bellman (1984) and Johansen (1996) both have found that secrets are not necessarily completely unknown to the uninitiated people of a community, but there are still ways of protecting the secret knowledge after it has been exposed to people who are not obligated to know. Johansen (p. 201) argues that to be taken seriously as a bearer of the esoteric knowledge held by Makonder men and women in Tanzania, Africa, one must have a legitimate right to the knowledge. She argues that a certain leakage can strengthen the secret, as the threat of punishment for revealing it clearly marks the borderline between open and concealed knowledge. However, one can never know if one has insight into the whole secret, and thus it seems impossible to penetrate the boundaries.

This corresponds with my findings in the Marka villages that the borders between what could be shared and what could not be shared with uninitiated people were rather flexible. If any part of the traditional healing knowledge is revealed to people who are not supposed to have access, there is still a way to protect the status of the knowledge as secret. There is a belief that if the written healing instructions come into the hands of the wrong people, they cannot be read or used. This was illustrated in the story at the beginning of this chapter in which a woman found her father's healing instructions and was prevented from reading them by a force that she interpreted as her deceased father. These written healing instructions were later lost, and there are different theories in the family as to where they disappeared. Nonetheless, the family was not worried that they had come into the hands of the wrong people, because it was believed that the inscriptions could not be used by anyone who had not been taught the knowledge or was not supposed to have it.

Another way of maintaining the secret is illustrated by a story told by a young woman who had once heard a healing formula when she was taken as a child to a *guvhllár*:

> When I was about seven or eight years old, my mom and I went to a *guvhllár*. She had to wait outside while the *guvhllár* and I went to

the kitchen. We talked a bit before he poured a glass of water from the tap, held his hand over the glass, and read something. And I was thinking that when I get out I am going to tell Mom what he read, because those were just regular words; it was not anything mystical. But the words were blown away, from the minute I walked out the kitchen door. I did not remember a word, not one!

The conclusion of this story was stated by a member of her family as follows: "If you hear those words, they are supposed to be forgotten; they are not intended to be remembered." This way of holding the formulas secret was also recounted in another story, in which a woman had been invited as a child to assist a *guvhllár*. The *guvhllár* had rejected her mother for the mission, explaining that a child was more suitable for the task. The girl heard the formula being read out loud but was told by the *guvhllár* that she was not supposed to remember it. And she did not.

The healing power of the knowledge is accordingly connected to a special approval for using it, and knowledge that is revealed without authorization loses its status. This is a way of discounting the status of the secret knowledge that is exposed, which was also found by Bellman (1984, pp. 48–49) in secret societies in West Africa. Bellman states that the medicine knowledge of the Zo is connected to an inherited ability or right to know, which also prevents it from being stolen. When a new person is going to be initiated into Zo medicine knowledge, important medicine leaves have to be informed that this person has the right to know and that they must work for him, before he is taught the particular rituals for picking the leaves.

Flexible Borders Between the Secret and the Open

Harrison (1995) elaborates on Barth's theory about the principles in the management of guru and conjurer knowledge, arguing that knowledge management is about balancing restriction and circulation. Both too much and too little openness around knowledge would be destructive to its value. Among the Manambu people in New Guinea he found that religious knowledge was generally held to be esoteric knowledge because the knowledge was significant for justifying their land rights, and if other clans gained insight into it, they could use it to claim title over Manambu land. The knowledge could still not be held too secret, because outsiders would have to know at least part of it in order to acknowledge it as a legitimate basis for claiming rights. The knowledge also had to be shared with a few outsiders in order to prevent it from being lost in case the older possessors of the knowledge passed away.

I have similar experiences with Sámi traditional healing knowledge. The borders between what is held in secret and what uninitiated people have insight into is not fixed, as shown by the fact that I was given different responses when I asked the holders of traditional healing knowledge for interviews. Even if there is a general norm against revealing traditional healing knowledge and claiming to have healing abilities, there are uninitiated persons who have actually received insight into relatively deep information about traditional healing practices. This line between the secret and the open can be stretched both ways, and the amount of knowledge that holders are willing to reveal about these things seems to depend on, among other things, the local tradition, the person who is asking, and the person who is being asked. The existence of geographical differences seemed to be evident when I discussed this with Sámi people from other areas and with other researchers who had studied traditional healing. I believe that the local tradition of secrecy is shaped by a range of factors, including religion, the history of the area, and the contact between different ethnic groups. Different individuals would probably also be approached differently, depending on the person's intentions for asking, whether he or she was considered a reliable person, and whether the person was an insider or an outsider.

What I found interesting during my fieldwork, however, was that individual possessors of knowledge responded in different ways to me as a researcher and seemed to have different limits for openness around these matters. Some of them talked relatively openly about their practice and convictions, while others were unwilling to indicate anything about their healing abilities. It seems, however, that openness was tolerated more from those traditional healers whose position was widely recognized and who had for some time clearly proven themselves worthy of their special abilities. With a stable position as a traditional healer they can allow themselves to stretch the rules further before the users start questioning their motives for this. They probably also have more self-confidence and trust that they know how much they can say; in addition, the users have more confidence in the healer's ability to evaluate how much can be revealed.

Mathisen (2000) suggests that these old norms connected to traditional medicine are gradually changing as the traditional medicine system is adapting to modern society, in which the media and technical communication play an important role. He observes that some therapists of traditional medicine promote to a greater degree their services in the newspaper and give interviews about their practices to the media. He considers that this new form of publicity exhibits continuity with the "great" traditional healers who were widely renowned from the oral narratives about them. He warns against creating the image of an overly "authentic" and static traditional medicine and argues that the values on which traditional medicine builds will be adapted to the contemporary reality. In the Marka villages I found that the secrecy norm was still highly relevant and that traditional healing was still surrounded by many taboos regarding how *guvhllárs* should behave and how they should relate to the special knowledge into which they had been initiated. The beliefs about the consequences of breaking these rules are still present, and the knowledge is still seen as being of such a character that not everyone can handle it.

The people to whom I spoke in the Marka villages hold the values that have been handed down by previous generations, but it is likely that not everyone in the villages is socialized identically into the same norms and values connected to traditional healing. The taboos were also vague or non-existent when it came to alternative medicine. Although some informants rejected alternative treatment as "humbug," there were also informants of all ages who were open to alternative treatment like acupuncture, homeopathy, and reiki healing. The growing popularity and recognition of alternative medicine in society at large is also mirrored in the Marka villages. People are open to trying new treatment methods, and those who are using alternative medicine seem to accept that there are different rules in this sector than in traditional medicine. To some degree, the norms and values concerning traditional healing do colour the way in which people look upon alternative therapists. As these therapists represent a tradition from the outside, I believe that they will continue to be evaluated on a more neutral ground and not in the same way as the local traditional healers. How this will be experienced in the future has yet to be seen. It will be interesting to see whether the values in alternative medicine will have an increasing influence on traditional healing.

Notes

1. These kinds of texts with healing instructions, remedies, and formulas are locally called *læsinga* (the readings) and are usually passed down through generations of traditional healers.

2. In the UNESCO *Convention for the Safeguarding of the Intangible Cultural Heritage* (2003), *safeguarding* is explained as the measures aimed at ensuring the viability of the intangible cultural heritage, including the identification, documentation, research, preservation, protection, promotion, enhancement, and transmission, particularly through formal and non-formal education, as well as the revitalization of the various aspects of such heritage.

3. The *noaidi* is explained by Bäckman (1988) as the spiritual leader of the old Sámi communities who had the ability to go into a trance and to communicate with gods and the spiritual world. The tasks of these leaders included obtaining information from distant places, locating lost items or reindeer, and engaging deceased descendants for herding the reindeer. The *noaidi* could foresee the future, find which god demanded what kind of sacrifice, and act as a leader in the sacrificing ceremonies. The *noaidi* also had the role of a doctor or a healer in diagnosing and treating sick people.

4. Snåsamannen ("the man from Snåsa") is a well-known traditional healer from Snåsa in Trøndelag, who is believed to have helped thousands of people during 50 years of practice. The publishing of his biography in 2008 provoked an extensive media debate in Norway about traditional healing and alternative medicine.

References

Bäckman, L. (1988). Noajdiens initiation. In J.I. Eriksen & H. Persson (Eds.), *Samisk shamanism* (pp. 58–74). Uppsala: Vattumannen Förlag.

Barth, F. (1994). *Manifestasjon og prosess*. Oslo: Universitetsforlaget.

Bellman, B.L. (1984). *The language of secrecy: Symbols & metaphores in Poro ritual*. New Brunswick, NJ: Rutgers University Press.

Blix Hagen, R. (2005). *Samer er trollmenn i norsk historie*. Karasjok, Norway: Čálliid lágádus.

Hætta, A.K. (2010). *Secret knowledge: The management and transformation of traditional healing knowledge in the Marka Sámi villages* (Master's thesis). University of Tromsø, Faculty of Social Science, Norway.

Hanem, T. (1999). Kartlegging av nokre folkelege førestellingar om sjukdom, død og ulukke i eir Samisk område: Drøfting av kliniske implikasjoner i møte med vestlig psykologi. Kautokeino, Nordisk samisk institutt, Dieđut 4/1999.

Hansen, L.I., and B. Olsen. (2004). *Samenes historie fram til 1750.* Oslo: Cappelsens forlag.

Harrison, S. (1995). Anthropological perspectives: On the management of knowledge. *Anthropology Today, 11*(5) (October, 1995), 10-14.

Johansen, R.E. (1996). Kunnskapsforvaltning og makt i et kjønnsperspektiv: En analyse av maskens hemmelighet. *Norsk Antropologisk tidsskrift, 3* (1996), 193-208.

Lov om alternativ behandling av sykdom mv. av 27. juni 2003 nr 64. [Act 64 of 27 June 2003 relating to the alternative treatment of disease, illness, etc.]. Oslo: Ministry of Health and Care Services. https://lovdata.no/dokument/NL/lov/2003-06-27-64 (accessed October 6, 2010).

Mathisen, S.R. (1983). *"Det er forskjell på folk og finner": En analyse av etnisk kategorisering i fortellertradisjonen* (Master's thesis). Universitetet i Bergen, Etno-folkloristisk institutt.

Mathisen, S.R. (2000): Folkemedisin i Nord-Norge: Kulturelt fellesskap og etniske skiller. In I. Altern & G. Minde (Eds.), *Samisk folkemedisin i dagens Norge* (pp. 15-34). Tromsø: Universiteteti Tromsø, Senter for samiske studier, Skriftsserie Nr. 9.

Miller, B.H. (2007). *Connecting and correcting: A case study of Sami healers in Porsanger.* Leiden, Netherlands: CNWS Publications.

Minde, G.T. (2000). Oppsummering av debatten. In I. Altern & G. Minde (Eds.), *Samisk folkemedisin i dagens Norge* (pp. 15-34). Tromsø: Universiteteti Tromsø, Senter for samiske studier, Skriftsserie Nr. 9.

Myrvoll, M. (2000). Kunnskapstradisjon og samiske helbredere. In I. Altern & G. Minde (Eds.), *Samisk folkemedisin i dagens Norge* (pp. 35-46). Tromsø: Universiteteti Tromsø, Senter for samiske studier, Skriftsserie Nr. 9.

Myrvoll, M. (2009). Knowledge traditions and healers in Sami society. (Lecture.) Presented on February 9 in HEL-3051, "Health Issues in an Indigenous Perspective with a Special Focus on Sami People," Faculty of Medicine, University of Tromsø.

Nergård, J.I. (2006). *Den levende erfaring: En studie i samisk kunnskapstradisjon.* Oslo: Cappelen akademisk forlag.

Rydving, H. (1995). *The end of drum time: Religious change among the Lule Saami, 1670s-1740s.* Uppsala: Uppsala University.

Sexton, R.H., & Buljo Stabbursvik, E.A. (2010). Healing in the Sámi north. *Culture, Medicine, and Psychiatry, 34*(4), 571-589.

Simmel, G. (1950). *The sociology of Georg Simmel.* (K.H. Wolff, Ed.). Free Press: New York.

Steen, A. (1961). Samenes folkemedisin. In A. Nesheim (Ed.), *Samiske samlinger bind V.* Oslo: Universitetsforlaget.

United Nations Education, Scientific, and Cultural Organization. (2003). *Convention for the safeguarding of the intangible cultural* heritage.

VG Nett. (2008, November 20). Snåsamannen: Har hjulpet 50.000 mennesker gratis. Ny bok om trønderen med de spesielle evnene trykt i 50.000 eksemplarer. Retrieved on October 6, 2010, from VG Nett website: www.vg.no/rampelys/ artikkel.php?artid=534115.

Weber, M. (2005): *Makt og byråkrati: Essay om politikk og klasse, samfunnsforskning og verdier.* Oslo: Gyldendal.

World Health Organization. (2005): *National policy on traditional medicine and regulation of herbal medicine.* (Report of a WHO global survey.) Geneva: World Health Organization.

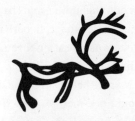

3

Traditional Sámi Healing
Heritage and Gifts of Grace

MARIT MYRVOLL

This chapter examines traditional Sámi healing as it is understood and practised by both users and practitioners living in a local community in Sápmi. There will be a special focus on the continuity and change in transmission and management of knowledge, as well as the villagers' use of healers (Myrvoll, 2011).[1]

Practitioners and users of traditional healing are as two sides of a coin—they cannot be separated. The users are dependent on a healer, and the healer is dependent on the people's need for her or him. It is the use of the healer that keeps the tradition alive and makes the popular health sector (Kleinman, 1980) user controlled. It also makes the healer, as well as the user, embedded in the same understanding and world view. Visible in what is made explicit and in what is implicit, they share the perceptions of who the healer is and why he or she became one. An example of the spectrum—the active user and the perceptions on healing and healer—is presented here with regard to a toothache.

Background

The data material concerns a Sámi community located on the coast of Northern Norway.[2] Måsske is a village of about 90 inhabitants, and the Sámi language, as well as Norwegian, is an everyday language, in both the private and the public arena. The name Måsske means a location through which there is no passage; you must turn around and go back the same way you came. This is a revealing description, Måsske being surrounded by high mountain peaks, most of which are about 1,000 metres above sea level. The deepest cave of northern Europe, Råggejávrrerájgge, is in one of these mountains. Owing to the high peaks, the sun is not seen for about three months every winter. Måsske is located in a coastal municipality characterized by its many fjords, and from the head of the longest fjord it is only six kilometres to the Swedish border. The village has no road connection to the outside world. The hydrofoil calls 11 times a week. In addition every family has at least one privately owned boat so that they can move independently of the regular service. The children learn how to cope with the sea at an early age. The fjord is the only, and the most important, means of communication. People in Måsske live from fishing, farming, woodcutting, and different kinds of service industry, often in various combinations. There is a high degree of awareness about living in Måsske; most inhabitants have made a deliberate choice in this regard.

Måsske is a village dominated by pietistic Christian belief, and the dogma and values of the Laestadian First Born Congregation[3] characterize daily life. The traditional Sámi healers referred to in the following are all pietistic Christians. Pietism spread from Germany in the seventeenth century and achieved great influence among Lutheran churches in Western Europe in the eighteenth century. When the Christian missionary work among the Sámi people started in the eighteenth century, it was led by the priest and pietist Thomas von Westen. The Laestadian movement has many pietistic hallmarks because it was designed as a pietistic movement—both in organization and in dogma—by its founder, Lars Levi Laestadius (Læstadius, 1997, pp. 341–392). The central emphasis is on conversion and repentance, remission of sins, and grace. Laestadius himself was a priest within the church, but he emphasized the importance of laymen being preachers. Through this practice he empowered the preaching of the faith and made a strong division between believers and non-believers. Laestadianism started in the mid-1800s as a mainly Sámi revival, but today the Sámi are a numerical minority (Bolle, 2000).

The Congregation Hall is located in the centre of the village. The congregation is important to people and functions as a centre for identification and confirmation of many fundamental common values, for conduct and behaviour. Only a minority of the adults are actual members of the congregation, but almost everyone in the village attends the services and raises their children by the values preached in the sermons. Life and reality is, however, more than the Congregation Hall. Religious reality is a diversity of matters that touches upon most aspects of life (Berger & Luckmann, 1966/2000; Geertz, 1973/1993a). The local world view is also composed of folk religious aspects, which open up dimensions that cannot be experienced in the same way as everyday reality but nevertheless are felt to exist, and people have to learn to manage them. Examples include experiences in connection with death or the phenomena of the underworld known as the little people. Health is also a field that people have to manage, and the use of traditional medicine is part of their strategies for the "good life." In summary, folk religious conceptions and practice appear as integral parts of the world view, and the world view expresses additionally that the god of Christianity is omnipotent.

In Måsske, as well as the surrounding society, the Sámi term *låhkke* is used for a traditional healer. In English it can be translated as "reader."[4] In this chapter I will use the term *healer* or *traditional healer*. When people say that they have been *read on*, it means that they have received healing from a traditional healer for a somatic illness, another kind of torment, or the prevention of illness or bad happenings.

The term *låhkåt* (to read, which is what the healer does) is said to have its origin in the fact that the traditional healer is supposed to have, and use, secret written formulas. However, also owing to tradition, the acquirement of such formulas is not the most important characteristic, because a person without the special spiritual powers and ability will never be able to help others. A variety of terms can refer to a healer, but, whatever the name referring to the traditional Sámi healer (both today and down through history), a healer has access to the knowledge that is inaccessible to others.

Traditional healers are careful not to compete with the doctors of school medicine. They always ask their patients if they have seen the doctor, or they encourage the patients to seek help from the school medicine sector. This practice has to be understood in relation to Norwegian legislation. Norway enacted a special penal code in 1936 forbidding all non-professionals to cure illnesses. This penal code was revoked after 67 years in 2004 and replaced by a new law allowing for alternative medicine. In other words, the traditional healer's practice was an offence under criminal law until 2004 when Norway enacted an act relating to the alternative treatment of disease, illness, etc.[5] Taking into account, on one side, the continuity of traditional healing and, on the other side, the change in the authorities' policy, it can be argued that it is the users of the folk sector of the health-care systems that have caused the change. Without users, there is no need for healers.

Toothache

In the beginning of August the whole school (all the pupils), many parents, and other adults, as well as pupils' younger siblings, went for a good week of hiking in the inland mountains, which are in Sweden. It was a journey taken in the footsteps of the forebears of the pupils. We moved in a landscape that had been used for both economic activity and communication. In my tent one night, upon going to bed, one of the girls, Therese, was tormented by an aching tooth. The other two girls lay down as well in pure solidarity. I asked Therese for her full name and date of birth before I started to search the big camp for a traditional healer. After six months of fieldwork in the village I thought I knew of five persons in the camp who were healers. I found that most people were in the big *lavvo*.[6] When I asked for help, the discussion started. One of the known traditional healers refused to help. He claimed that to take away the girl's toothache would be a disservice because the pain would be forever gone and the teeth would rot in her mouth. He reminded everyone that dentists had been angry with healers because of this. Many others disagreed and said that this was a special situation because we were located far up in the mountains and there were no dentists around. He still refused. Despite this discussion many people came to our tent, and to my knowledge at least three healers were among them. The next morning they returned and made Therese promise to see a dentist when she went home. For the remaining days of the hike Therese did not complain. Her toothache had gone.

Prior to our departure for the hike one of the adults had told me that everyone should bring a first-aid kit with them in case something unexpected happened. It was said that the first-aid kit should include competence in coping with unwanted experiences. The healing competence should include the ability to relieve pain and to stop bleeding—whether it be small or copious. In addition, one should bring competence in *suonav tjadnat* (Sámi for "to tie the tendon") in case one missteps and strains a foot. Bringing pure woollen yarn and a knife was mandatory in case of accidents or illness. However, this person never did tell me how to use the knife or the yarn or where to obtain the necessary competence.

I do not know whether all this competence was present during the eight-day-long hike. What I thought I knew, after having lived in the village for over six months, was who were and who were not the traditional healers. None of them had actually told me. I would ask, "Are there any traditional healers in the village?" The individual always named someone else, never himself or herself. With this information, however, I was able to take action when Therese was troubled by her toothache. I was also told that toothache was one of the most difficult pains to cure.

Culture, World View, and Health

The comprehension of good health and a good life is subject to cultural perspectives (Olsen & Eide, 1999), as are other areas such as happiness, luck, beauty, and wealth. The understanding of health depends on the understanding of illness, and health-care systems are socially and culturally constructed and differ from culture to culture and society to society. Kleinman (1980, pp. 49-60) considers health as a holistic cultural system, and he refers to Berger and Luckmann's (1966/2000) perspective when he states that "health care systems are socially and culturally constructed. They are forms of social reality" (Kleinman, 1980, p. 35). He says that in the same way as religion, language, or kinship are looked upon as cultural systems, the field of medicine is a corresponding system: "a system of symbolic meanings anchored in particular arrangements of social institutions and patterns of interpersonal interactions" (p. 24). According to Kleinman, the medical and health field includes people's perception of illness as well as the possibilities and methods for a cure. In this way, perceptions of health would not be understood apart from people's practice in the field of health. Such a perspective is closely related to Geertz's (1973/1993) definition of a cultural system as a "model for" and a "model of" behaviour because both the perceptions and the practice constitute health as a system.

The World Health Organization defines health as "a state of complete physical, mental, and social well-being and not merely the absence of disease or infirmity."[7] The definition states that physical health as well as mental health and the social surroundings of a person are important for the total health situation. Health is often viewed by indigenous peoples as being dependent upon the appropriate relationship between the individual and the community. This view is supported by the Aboriginal and Torres Strait Islander Health Council in Australia, which states that, for Australian aboriginal people, health is not only about the absence of illness or about access to doctors, hospitals, and medicines but predominantly about being able to cope with one's life, including the physical environment and one's own norms for dignity, respect, self-confidence, and social justice. Hereby the focus is on both physical health and mental health, as well as on social and emotional well-being (NATSIHC, 2003, pp. 2–3).

"Good life" is closely connected with spirituality and religion in many societies, and therefore health and world view are seen in relation to religious perceptions. The view of what constitutes good life has to do with external influences and circumstances—like managing different situations—and with internal perceptions connected to values and world view. Religion becomes important to many because it offers explanations for the bad and the good conditions of life (see Klass, 1995, pp. 56–62). On the one hand, the believer knows from religious conviction the reason that suffering, illness, and death exist and is therefore not preoccupied with explaining these facts. On the other hand, the believer seeks explanations for isolated incidents, with questions such as "Why did my brother die?" "Why has the harvest gone bad this year?" For someone in crisis or in need, religion becomes increasingly important. Geertz (1973/1993, p. 104) says: "As a religious problem, the problem of suffering is, paradoxically, not how to avoid suffering but how to suffer, how to make of physical pain, personal loss, worldly defeat, or the helpless contemplation of others' agony something bearable, supportable—something, as we say, sufferable."

Religion gives thus an important explanation and offers purpose and a deeper sense of meaning to those in need or in pain because of their own or others' sufferings. The content of these explanations differs from religion to religion, but the need to give purpose to apparently meaningless situations seems to be universal (McGuire, 1992).

Traditional Medicine

In its definition of traditional medicine the World Health Organization (2005, p. 1) states: "Traditional Medicine has a long history. It is the sum total of the knowledge, skills, and practices based on the theories, beliefs, and experiences indigenous to different cultures, whether explicable or not, used in the maintenance of health as well as in prevention, diagnosis, improvement, or treatment of physical and mental illnesses."

Further, the World Health Organization divides the different medical fields into school medicine or Western medicine; alternative medicine; and traditional medicine. These are not precise fields, but they have to be understood in the context of where they are practised. For instance, traditional Chinese medicine (TCM) could be considered alternative when practised in Norway. In the same way, traditional Sámi medicine could be considered alternative when practised outside its Sámi context. Traditional and alternative medicine are considered by many to be alternative or complementary to school medicine. They are also diverse in their practices, and traditional medicine in Northern Norway is no exception, including as it does Sámi, Norwegian, and Kven treatment traditions (Mathisen, 2000).

Over time the Sámi people have developed their own traditional medicine, knowledge, and experiences about illnesses and sufferings and how to cure them. Johan Turi, the first Sámi writer of a Sámi book, *Muittalus samid birra* (Stories about the Sámi people), opens the chapter about healing by stating that he would not tell about all illnesses and ways to cure them, because *oahppan hearrat* (the scholarly men) would laugh at the Sámi way of healing (Turi, 1910/1965). This presumption from Turi probably arises from his knowledge about the way in which Sámi medicine was seen in contrast to school medicine by the main society, to quote Mathisen (2000, p. 15): "In much of what has been written about folk medicine, it is commonly described as a kind of contrast to the established school medicine—and is connected with a lack of common sense, irrationality, and superstition. The traditional is seen as in opposition to the modern, to science and enlightenment" (author's translation).

Kleinman (1980) thinks that, when someone falls ill, the Western biomedical model does not take into account the aspect of meaning. He developed his theoretical framework for an ethno medical model because he felt that the biomedical model was too influenced by Western cultural perceptions. To Kleinman, a Western theoretical and value-based perspective pervaded the biomedical model, and therefore the latter did not take into consideration the patient's perspectives on health and diseases. Furthermore, the Western model excluded the alternative treatment methods that are found in other societies and cultures. Kleinman wanted to develop "an ethno medical model that can systematically compare different culturally constituted frameworks for construing sickness" (1980, p. 18). In this model he differentiates between the concepts of illness and disease, in which illness is the patient's experience of his or her symptoms, and disease is the diagnosis from the doctor (Ingstad, 2007, p. 43). In the meeting between patient and doctor it is not evident that the patient receives a diagnosis that is understandable or that the doctor has the same frame of cultural understanding and references as the patient. Since Western school medicine more or less has had a monopoly when it comes to the diagnosis of diseases (supported by legislation), it is understandable that people have made choices, visiting the doctor for certain symptoms, and the traditional healer for illnesses that they feel he or she can help (Ingstad, 2007).

Mathisen (2000) has the same understanding and thinks that school medicine views illness as an isolated physiological phenomenon, while traditional medicine understands and explains illness in relation to social and cultural conditions. Certainly conceptions of illness should be seen in their connection to the world view. This understanding of illness also applies to Sámi traditional medicine. For instance, the cause of illness can be explained as the influence of powers that are external to the sick person. Mathisen points out that in old writings about illnesses there is a tendency to explain them as external powers influencing the human body (2000, p. 18). Another explanation according to Mathisen is that illnesses and pains can be due to a lack of balance in the human body. He gave bleeding as an example, whereby extensive and long-lasting bleeding has to be stopped in order for the body's balance to be restored.

Pain caused by surgery can also be stopped by external powers. Today, in the unusual case that the patient does not need painkillers after surgery, hospital personnel in Northern Norway will ask whether the patient had contacted a traditional healer. These hospitals have experienced that patients have less or no pain when a traditional healer has been involved. This does not change the medical diagnosis or treatment; the hospital staff just observes the patient's condition and wishes for information about the use of several health sectors. For the patient the question about the use of a traditional healer is regarded positively, otherwise without this question the general assumption is that the school medicine does not approve of the traditional one.

Open and Secret Knowledge

Traditional medicine among the Sámi people becomes in Kleinman's terminology a part of the folk sector of health care. Sámi traditional medicine, as well as folk medical traditions in other societies and cultures, is embedded in a different knowledge tradition than that of Western school medicine. Sámi healers are the keepers and managers of this knowledge. However, such a tradition of knowledge is not only connected to the healers as individuals. The healers are, at the same time, embedded in a larger context; they live and practise in geographical, social, and cultural communities. Everyone, both on an individual and on a collective level, is embedded in a historical and cultural context of practice, thinking, and doing, concerning either worldly matters or more sacral activities, which cannot be understood without seeing the interconnection of these activities in a wider context. It is important to note that healers' knowledge is locally accepted as esoteric, and only healers have the competence, insight, and responsibility for the management of this knowledge. This is expressly not an open and general knowledge to which everyone has access (Myrvoll, 2000).

The traditional healer is central in the folk sector of health, but this field comprises more than healing by spiritual abilities; it includes, for instance, herbs, minerals, food, and various ritual practices. Everybody can learn and practise how to remove a wart and how to use woollen yarn to remove pain. But there is an important dividing line in the management of traditional medicine, and it is drawn by tradition itself. Although the ability to stop bleeding is considered a competence that every family and household should have, this practice belongs to the traditional healer's competence and is thus looked upon as esoteric knowledge with the accompanying use of secret formulas. The formulas must be passed on from one generation of healers to the next and have to be used as they were originally intended. The healer has an obligation to respect the formulas that she or he has been given.

Historical Healing Practice

The modern Western medicine and health system does not have a long presence in the Sámi areas, and therefore we can look at changes in the societal infrastructure that have had an impact on the healers and their role in the Sámi society. Before public health districts were established in the nineteenth century, the priests (Christian) often took care of sick persons. As a religious professional, the priest took responsibility for the diagnosis, medicine, and treatment; this practice coincided with the role played by the noajdde[8] or shaman in the pre-Christian Sámi religion. Traditional Sámi healing is connected to the Sámi world view; the religion and world view within Sámi society has changed, and so has the understanding of traditional medicine and healing.

In the pre-Christian Sámi society when Sámi religion was practised, the noajdde was a religious expert and an adviser about the will of the gods, as well as being a ritual master with knowledge of the future and other hidden realities. The noajdde was also the most powerful healer, especially when serious illness occurred (Bäckman, 1987). Health and healing were thus closely connected to religion and world view, affirming a holistic view in which health was a relation between the individual and the community.

There were probably several persons in every local community who had knowledge about illnesses and how to cure them, but the noajdde would be contacted in the severe cases. Old manuscripts written by priests tell of the *noajdde* and his or her skills in healing. The general perception was that when a person fell ill, it was because someone, most likely a dead person, had stolen the soul of the sick one. The *noajdde* had to travel to the realm of the dead to negotiate the soul's return home (Pollan, 2002, pp. 69–74). The understanding of illness is connected to the perception that a soul can be lost or stolen by powers external to the sick person. The soul can also be damaged by objects under the control of an evil person (Kristiansen, 2005, p. 28). The *noajdde* had the competence to find the cause of the disease and had the knowledge about how or if it could be cured. She or he also had the ability to move between the visible and the invisible parts of reality, both to the realm of the gods and to the realm of the dead. In these realms the *noajdde* needed the skills to negotiate the best outcome for individuals and the community.

When the Christian missionaries and priests came to Sápmi in the eighteenth century, they probably looked for religious experts similar to themselves and discovered the male *noajdde* as the main target of their cause, the change of beliefs. Perhaps they did not see, or bother about, the healing activities and tasks. Their main focus was the introduction of the Christian religion and world view, which included the consequences of eternal life in heaven or hell. The Sámi healing institution survived the change to Christianity, although it was practised within a different world view.

The forbidding of Sámi healing and medicine by law has a long history in Norway. The first Christian laws in Norway (made before 1120) are Eidsivatingsloven and Borgartingsloven, and they were made for the population of southeastern Norway. The laws had five clauses about the Sámi all relating to the prohibition of contacting a Sámi for help when a distress had been caused by sorcery (Hansen & Olsen, 2004, p. 108). On the one hand, this shows that there must have been Sámi settlements in the south of Norway, and, on the other hand, it reveals very clearly the Norwegian or Norse society's view of the Sámi.

The *noajdde* as they have been described in the old manuscripts have gone. Pollan (1993) claims that the end of Sámi shamanism as a cultural phenomenon was caused by Christian missionary work. The changes in religious belief and practice from the Sámi religion to Christianity became too extensive. At the same time, Sámi communities needed healers. The missionary work and change in religion came far ahead of any modern society's health-care system into the Sámi areas, and although the function as religious expert and ritual master ended, the function as healer continued and still exists.

The missionaries' aim was to Christianize the Sámi population. All the religious aspects that they interpreted as non-Christian beliefs and rituals were considered the devil's work. The Sámi religion thus became demonized. The *noajdde* was looked upon as a tool of the devil, and the Sámi religious practice was defined as evil. The missionaries' main intention was to put an end to the Sámi religious beliefs as well as to the authority of the *noajdde*. They probably did not attach importance to the healer function of the *noajdde*. As long as the Sámi stopped invoking their old gods in a ritual context, the missionary work was considered successful.

There are no descriptions of the way in which the process of change affected healing work, no tracking of its move as a social institution from Sámi religion to Christianity. It has probably been a long process, connected to the appointment and initiating steps as well as to the local use of the *noajdde*. The Sámi healing institution today is an integrated part of the Christian cultural heritage and bears witness to an extensive capacity for adaption and survival. It also shows how strong the interdependence must have been between the local community and the *noajdde* as a healer. The healer understood the importance of bringing the healing knowledge down through the generations, while the local community used and protected the healing institution. Its existence was not revealed to the majority society. And then, later, owing to Norwegian legislation, it became necessary to keep the tradition silent (Myrvoll, 2000).

Present Traditional Healing

My main point has been that Sámi healers, past and present, cannot be practitioners of healing without users. People's use of healers and the need for healing keep the tradition alive. It makes the folk sector of health (Kleinman, 1980) a user-controlled sector. The ancient *noajdde*, the current traditional healer, and the Sámi neo-shaman have in common that there are human needs underlying their practice (Myrvoll, 2000). Down through time the *noajdde* and most of the Christian traditional healers have lived in communities where they have practised their skills. Some healers are known far beyond their communities and receive many requests for assistance via the telephone. Before the telephone was common, people wrote letters to the healers or came from afar to seek help for their illness. Mathisen (2000) has described the practice of a famous healer, Johannes Brateng (1890–1967), who was himself affected by cerebral palsy. Brateng was a Christian, and it is said that he had experienced God giving him the choice to become healthy or to have the ability to heal others. He chose the latter, and countless sick people visited him in his home. It was not uncommon for him to treat 70–80 people in a day (Mathisen, 2000, p. 21).

A visit to a healer can make a lasting impression. A woman in the Måsske village told of an experience that she had had as a nine-year-old. Her parents had taken her to a healer to cure a problem with her adenoids. She remembers that the healer had a little key that he twisted around outside her neck. He asked her to open her mouth, and it seemed to her as a little girl that the healer spat into her mouth. She was so offended that she washed out her mouth several times. As an adult she realized that the healer had blown on her and that this had given rise to the misunderstanding and insult she had felt. This narrative describes the use of multiple medical sectors. Probably the parents of the child had taken her first to the local doctor, who had diagnosed the adenoids condition. What had made her parents decide to see a healer instead of pursuing further treatment in the public health sector was not known. Maybe the school-medicine diagnosis was such that an operation was not recommended. The parents sought the folk sector of health in the form of a healer whom they knew. According to the woman, she had no more problems after the healer's treatment.

Healing is not a uniform field. In some families such abilities can be distributed among siblings or cousins: a sister or a brother can be clairvoyant; another can have dreams that foretell the future; and then a third can be a strong healer who has both—clairvoyance and dreams that foretell the future. Some families are considered more important carriers of healing traditions than others. Healers can be considered strong or less strong, in the sense that all do not have an equal ability to create relief or improvement in sick people. Some are considered good at "taking" inflammation, others at relieving toothache or pain. Some are masters who "bind" the tendon or stop the blood. And, as has been said, others have a reputation for being clairvoyant and having dreams that foretell the future. A healer who has all these abilities is often considered strong enough to turn around hopeless cases. It was told about a healer from the village who was so strong that he could awaken people from a coma.

Stories about healers are usually told during talk about completely different issues. If I tried to bring up the subject, it was usually laughed away. It seemed to be culturally unacceptable to talk too much about healers who lived and worked in the community. As the story about the toothache testifies, I did become familiar with some of the practices associated with the healing institution in the community. I spoke with many people who were considered to be healers or to have special abilities, although healing as a theme was rarely touched upon. In my experience, it was almost impossible to get a healer to mention his or her own abilities. I perceived that anyone regarded as a healer would actually pull away from the social arena when the conversation touched upon the subject. The reaction was different, however, when a healer was asked for help. Then the seeker was defined as someone in need, recognizing the healer's capability to help.

Only one of the traditional healers in the local community talked to me about his competence and his practice. He believed that "basically a traditional healer may heal all kinds of ailments and diseases. It is most common to heal pain and inflammation, and also stop blood and blood poisoning. Recently it is also more and more common to heal people's mental disorders such as anxiety. A healer is able to send away ghosts if someone is bothered by them. The healer can also heal a person's general life, for example by giving protection or sending away afflictions or plagues" (author's translation).

What the traditional healer tells is consistent with the villagers' view on traditional healing practice. Today it is common to contact a traditional healer before giving birth or taking an exam. The traditional healer is believed to be able to "ease" forthcoming hardships.

People perceived the healer's abilities as coming from two different but equal origins: inheritance and Christian gifts of grace. Inherited abilities pass from parents to children, from mother or father to daughter or son. The abilities can also skip a generation, passing from grandmother or grandfather to grandchild, or can pass from aunt or uncle to niece or nephew. If a child does not want to take on the abilities, it will not be exposed to pressure. The giving of the abilities to the younger generation may have its origin in the tradition that a traditional healer should not teach someone older than himself or herself. If the healer does so, the healer will lose the powers, according to the tradition.

Christian gifts of grace are mentioned in the Bible. The summons was made in the words of Jesus to his disciples: "Heal the sick, raise the dead, cleanse those who have leprosy, drive out demons. Freely you have received; freely give" (Matthew 10:8). This verse not only legitimizes the continuation of traditional healers but also provides a clear direction that a healer cannot claim compensation for using the healing abilities, not even a simple "thank you" from the patients. In the village there is a strong tradition of never thanking a healer, because the healing powers would be lost. This is an absolute rule because it is believed that healing comes from God. The traditional healer is certainly not God, just an instrument of God's power.

At one point in a conversation about the origin of healing powers a Bible was placed on the table, and reference was made to the Book of Luke: "The seventy-two returned with joy and said, 'Lord, even the demons submit to us in your name.' He replied, 'I saw Satan fall like lightning from heaven. I have given you authority to trample on snakes and scorpions and to overcome all the power of the enemy; nothing will harm you. However, do not rejoice that the spirits submit to you, but rejoice that your names are written in heaven'" (Luke 10:17–20). Here, as in several other verses in the Bible, reference is made to the spirits as powers external to man, powers that have to obey the disciples. This is a perception coinciding largely with a world view that diseases and other problems can be caused by forces external to a person. Miller (2007, pp. 240–241) writes from a Sámi community (Porsanger) further north in Norway that within traditional Sámi healing, concepts like "binding" or "loosing" illnesses or ailments are used. These are concepts that would otherwise be used within Laestadian terminology for the process of forgiveness, and Miller believes that this shows how integrated traditional healing is with Laestadianism.

The relationship between God's gifts and the healer's abilities is generally accepted. Christians in the Laestadian congregation have great knowledge of the Bible, and in conversations on this matter reference was also made to Paul's first letter to the Corinthians concerning Christian gifts of grace:

There are different kinds of gifts, but the same Spirit distributes them. There are different kinds of service, but the same Lord. There are different kinds of working, but in all of them and in everyone it is the same God at work. Now to each one the manifestation of the Spirit is given for the common good. To one there is given through the Spirit a message of wisdom, to another a message of knowledge by means of the same Spirit, to another faith by the same Spirit, to another gifts of healing by that one Spirit, to another miraculous powers, to another prophecy, to another distinguishing between spirits, to another speaking in different kinds of tongues, and to still another the interpretation of tongues. (1 Corinthians 12:4–10)

The Bible verses emphasize that within Christianity the healer is appointed by God—just as in pre-Christian Sámi religion the *noajdde* is appointed by powers from outside. The healer is also defined by his or her heritage. To be a traditional healer is to receive both an inheritance from parents or another close relative, and the gift from God. Mathisen (2000, p. 20) writes: "In the traditional stories about people with healing abilities, this is explained in two parallel ways. On the one hand, it is emphasized that these individuals are selected by the powers themselves, and, on the other hand, with inheritance the abilities are passed down within certain families" (author's translation).

A person from the village who practised as a healer told me that he had learned a few formulas from his father after he had had an experience of helping a close relative. Later he learned more, such as protecting himself against evil. Eventually he created his own formulas, and he said that he often prayed while in meditation. In addition, he dreamt of coming deaths or other dramatic events. He had not yet experienced the failure of a dream foretelling the future. He said of his experiences with healing:

When I think of healing, my hands get hot. It's all about concentration and focus. Sometimes I get hot hands without knowing what it is, but I do know that someone needs my help. Then I pray.... I use a knife when I have to send evil away from a house or room or place. Most elderly healers use a knife. Fire, steel, and God's word are equal in my opinion. Ghosts and underground people are afraid of all this. The devil is most afraid of God's word. When there is evil afoot, it is only God's word that is capable and strong enough. Often you have to heal several times in the same place or co-operate with other healers.

There are still traditional healers. Despite the laws against quacksalvers and there being a monopoly on disease treatment, the school medicine has not been able to change the understanding and put an end to all practice in traditional medicine. About their relationship Mathisen (2000, p. 27) says the following:

> Among the representatives of the official, scientific medicine, the unofficial treatment methods have been understood in terms of a lack of knowledge and an ignorance among the population. One result of this is that it was believed that the popular treatment would die out of its own accord when the information became more available to the common people. This has been the opinion for almost two centuries, but the popular treatment has shown to be remarkably tenacious in many different segments of the population. (Author's translation)

Today it seems that traditional medicine has greater legitimacy than it did just a few decades ago. There has been an apparent increase in the use of alternative treatment and alternative medicine, as well as an understanding that school medicine has its limitations. The fact that people report to a greater degree than before about their use of treatments other than school medicine (Altern, 2000) can also indicate that it has become more acceptable to talk about alternative medical care in recent years. Such reporting does not necessarily indicate that the number of users has increased.

The relationship between users and practitioners of traditional medicine is largely based on trust. The user seeks a healer in the hopes of a positive outcome, not to learn how the healer achieves results. One woman put it this way: "I believe in my experience." She said that she had no knowledge about school medicine, "doctor's business," or traditional Sámi "reading," but when she needed help, she looked for what worked for her, no matter the medical sector from which it came (Myrvoll, 2003, p. 227). The woman considered both modern health care and traditional healing as expert systems of knowledge. This is comparable to Giddens's (1990) description of abstract expert systems in modern society. According to Giddens, expert systems are one of the hallmarks of modernity because there are many of them and they are large in scope. International air travel can stand as an example. Passengers want to get from A to B, but they have no desire or need to familiarize themselves with the pilot's competence in flying large airplanes or with the extensive logistics behind a grid of all corresponding flights. Modern expert systems are so complex and inaccessible to the public that they can be compared to esoteric knowledge. The woman wants to be freed from her ailments when she seeks a medical expert—be it a doctor with a medical degree or a traditional healer. She has no intention of acquiring detailed knowledge of these systems, but she is confident that they will be of help when she needs it, even if the knowledge system is closed and unavailable to her. Users of traditional healers are aware that their healers or helpers manage an esoteric knowledge to which they will not have access.

Altern (2000, p. 1) points out in a discussion about knowledge and world view that "embedded in our notions of what can be done to alleviate or cure illnesses and diseases, there are also perceptions of the basic order of existence" (author's translation). Similar to Berger and Luckmann (1966/2000), Altern thinks that perceptions of reality are often taken for granted. People have lived for generations with various medical systems that are in great contrast to each other in terms of an interpretation of disease. This also applies to Måsske. I did not have the impression that the various medical systems created much of a dilemma for people. Many said that they never told the local doctor that they also sought help from a traditional healer. Diagnosis and healing were explained with a smile: "I see the doctor to find out what is wrong with me, and then I see a healer to get well." This is consistent with Kleinman's (1980) distinction between illness and disease (diagnosis) but also shows that healing—"recovery"—may be culturally determined. People do not reject the professional health-care sector but use it in addition; they use and integrate the popular sector actively into the healing process. If, for example, someone is tormented by a nosebleed, the simplest treatment is to seek a healer who can stop it. At the same time the patient concedes to not knowing whether the nosebleed will turn out to be a symptom of a serious illness. Therefore he or she sees a doctor "to find out what is wrong with me."

The people of Måsske distinguish clearly between traditional and alternative medicine, as well as between traditional and school medicine. In addition to individual prevention and treatment of illness, health and healing include three active systems in the village: school medicine, traditional medicine, and alternative medicine. These work side by side and are not mutually exclusive. However, it is necessary to clarify that there are parts of the alternative medicine sector that are not used by local inhabitants. This applies to the treatment offered by neo-shamans. The religious practice of neo-shamanism is considered by several inhabitants to be Satanism. According to Laestadians, neo-shamanism is an evil practice because it does not embrace Christianity. This attitude shows the intimate relationship between health, healing, and religious beliefs, and, of course, is similar to the attitude taken by the church toward Sámi religion in the 1700s, with a dualistic idea that Christianity is related to the good or the divine and that everything else is evil, and thus becomes demonized (Alver & Selberg, 1992).

Conclusion

This chapter has focused on some aspects of traditional healing and on the way it is understood and practised in Måsske, both as a traditional medical system and in relation to other medical systems. In their management of illness and disease the local people often integrate several medical systems, depending on what they define as their needs. Over time the Sámi people have developed their own traditional medicine, based on the knowledge of diseases and the experience of healing them. In addition to the knowledge of healing herbs and natural medicines, the Sámi use traditional healers. The essay has mainly focused on the Sámi traditional healer (*låhkke*) and how the healer is legitimized through selection and knowledge management.

According to Mathisen (2000), the practice of consulting traditional healers depends on cultural values: "When people are faced with a crisis situation as in a case of disease, current beliefs and values that people experience as fundamental are made relevant within a cultural context" (p. 28). Altern (2000) says that the users' needs are crucial to the continuous use of healers. Even though the knowledge of traditional healers has been reserved for the few, it has nevertheless been necessary as a part of the community's collective knowledge and expertise in the treatment of disease and other ailments. A healer, today as in former times, receives his or her calling from the spiritual and divine powers. In a Christian context the calling, or the abilities, is defined as coming directly from the Christian God and becomes realized through Bible verses about gifts of grace.

Similar to the Laestadian preacher, the traditional healer can be said to have some of the characteristics that Weber (1971) ascribes for the traditional and charismatic leader. A traditional rule is characterized by the belief that the arrangements and the ruling power have existed since ancient times and are sacred. Weber maintains patriarchy as the most genuine traditional supremacy in which the ruler is looked upon as sacred and worthy and is obeyed because of tradition. However, this has the consequence that the ruler is limited by tradition. If she or he violates the rules of tradition and the norms, the legitimacy of leadership is in danger. According to Weber (1971, p. 98), in contrast to the traditional rule, the charismatic domination is a rule by virtue and devotion to the person's gifts of grace (charisma). Traditional healing seems to be a very strict practice when it comes to selection and management of knowledge. A traditional healer has, of course, no status as a traditional leader; however, I believe that the selection is comparable with the way in which the traditional and charismatic leader is appointed. Inheritance and gifts of grace point respectively to traditional and charismatic leadership. Inheritance allows the healer institution to follow family lines and kinship, while gifts of grace are a charismatic trait, according to Weber (ibid.). The practitioner is bound by the tradition. If people do not perceive that the healer has received the abilities correctly, which is according to tradition, and is managing them correctly, they will cease to seek the healer. This was very evident in conversations about neo-shamans and their healing practice. Basically people did not doubt that a neo-shaman had healing capabilities, but these capabilities were managed incorrectly, that is incorrectly when set in a traditional understanding (Myrvoll, 2000). People in the village considered announcements in the media, general talk about oneself as a healer, or the demand of payment for healing to be contradictory to the tradition and its management. Anyone violating the tradition in this way would lose his or her legitimacy as a healer.

Being a traditional healer is a complicated matter. One of the villagers expressed it thus: "I know of no one who has become haughty or arrogant in their role as a traditional healer. If so, people will not use you anymore. It is in a way self-regulating."

Notes

1. The chapter is a shortened version of one of the chapters in my doctoral dissertation, "Bare gudsordet duger: Om kontinuitet og brudd i samisk virkelighetsforståelse" (Continuity and change in Sámi world view).
2. All facts about the village date from my fieldwork in 1999.
3. Laestadian First Born Congregation members proclaim their status as true followers of Laestadius's original message.
4. In other Sámi areas there are other Sámi and Norwegian terms, such as *guvhllár* and *buorideaddji* (in Sámi) and *kurerer* and *blåser* (in Norwegian).
5. https://lovdata.no/dokument/NL/lov/2003-06-27-64/§2#§2 (February 24, 2015).
6. *Lavvo* is a traditional Sámi tent, used as a mobile home.
7. Preamble to the Constitution of the World Health Organization as adopted by the International Health Conference, New York, June 19–July 22, 1946; signed on July 22, 1946, by the representatives of 61 States (Official Records of the World Health Organization, no. 2, p. 100) and entered into force on April 7, 1948. http://www. who.int/governance/eb/who_constitution_en.pdf?ua=1 (February 24, 2015).
8. *Noajdde* is a Lule-Sámi term; *noaidi* in northern Sámi. The *noajdde* could be either female or male—there are stories about both.

References

The Aboriginal and Torres Strait Islander Health Council. (2003). *National strategic framework for Aboriginal and Torres Strait Islander health.* [Prepared for the Australian Health Ministers' Conference in 2003]. Retrieved from http://www. naccho.org.au/download/naccho-historical/nsfatsihcont.pdf (accessed on February 24, 2015).

Act relating to the alternative treatment of disease, illness, etc. Retrieved from https://lovdata.no/dokument/NL/lov/2003-06-27-64/§2#§2 (accessed on February 24, 2015).

Altern, I. (2000). Innledning. In I. Altern & G.-T. Minde (Eds.), *Samisk folkemedisin i dagens Norge*, vol. 9 (pp. iv–103). Tromsø: Senter for samiske studier, Universitetet i Tromsø.

Alver, B.G., & Selberg, T. (1992). *Det er mer mellom himmel og jord: Folks forståelse av virkeligheten ut fra forestillinger om sykdom og behandling.* Sandvika, Norway: Vett & Viten.

Bäckman, L. (1987). The noaidie, the Sami shaman. In M.M. Jocelyne Fernandez-Vest (Ed.), *Kalevala et traditions orales du Monde: Colloques Internationaux du CNRS.* Paris: CNRS.

Bäckman, L. (1988). Hur blev man noajdie? In H. Persson (Ed.), *Samerna: Hot, motstånd, tradition* (pp. 34–45). Stockholm: Föreningen Fjärde Värden.

Berger, P.L., & Luckmann, T. (1966/2000). *Den samfunnsskapte virkelighet.* Bergen: Fagbokforlaget.

The Bible. [New international version]. Retrieved from http://www.biblegateway.com (accessed on February 24, 2015).

Bolle, R. (2000). Læstadianismen i det moderne samfunnet. In Ø. Norderval & S. Nesset (Eds.),*Vekkelse og vitenskap: Lars Levi Læstadius 200 år, Ravnetrykk* (pp. 139–156). Tromsø: Universitetsbiblioteket i Tromsø.

Geertz, C. (1973/1993). *The interpretation of cultures: Selected essays.* London: Fontana.

Giddens, A. (1990). *The consequences of modernity.* Cambridge: Polity Press.

Hansen, L.I., & Olsen, B. (2004). *Samenes historie fram til 1750.* Oslo: Cappelen Akademisk Forlag.

Ingstad, B. (2007). *Medisinsk antropologi: En innføring.* Bergen: Fagbokforlaget.

Klass, M. (1995). *Ordered universes: Approaches to the anthropology of religion.* Boulder, CO: Westview Press.

Kleinman, A. (1980). *Patients and healers in the context of culture: An exploration of the borderland between anthropology, medicine, and psychiatry.* Berkeley: University of California Press.

Kristiansen, R. (2005). *Samisk religion og læstadianisme.* Bergen: Fagbokforlaget.

Læstadius, L.L. (1997). *Dårhushjonet: En blick i nådens ordning; systematiskt framställd under form af betracktelser öfwer själens egenskaper och tillstånd.* Skellefteå, Sweden: Artos.

Mathisen, S.R. (2000). Folkemedisinen i Nord-Norge: Kulturelt fellesskap og etniske skiller. In I. Altern & G.-T. Minde (Eds.), *Samisk folkemedisin i dagens Norge*, vol. 9 (pp. 15–33). Tromsø: Senter for samiske studier, Universitetet i Tromsø.

McGuire, M.B. (1992). *Religion: The social context.* Belmont, CA: Wadsworth Thomson Learning.

Miller, B.H. (2007). *Connecting and correcting: A case study of Sami healers in Porsanger.* Leiden, Netherlands: Research School CNWS, Universiteit Leiden.

Myrvoll, M. (2000). Kunnskapstradisjon og samiske helbredere. In I. Altern & G.-T. Minde (Eds.), *Samisk folkemedisin i dagens Norge*, vol. 9 (pp. 35–46). Tromsø: Senter for samiske studier, Universitetet i Tromsø.

Myrvoll, M. (2003). Old Age eller New Age: Nyreligiøsitet i det samiske samfunnet. In T. Lund-Olsen & P. Repstad (Eds.), *Forankring eller frikobling? Kulturperspektiver på religiøst liv i dag* (pp. 227–232). Bergen: Høyskoleforlaget.

Myrvoll, M. (2011). *"Bare gudsordet duger": Om kontinuitet og brudd i samisk virkelighetsforståelse*. Institutt for arkeologi og sosialantropologi, Universitetet i Tromsø.

NIFAB. Retrieved from http://www.nifab.no/ (accessed on September 14, 2012).

Olsen, T., & Eide, A. K. (1999). *"Med ei klype salt": Håndtering av helse og identitet i en flerkulturell sammenheng*. Bodø, Norway: Nordlandsforskning.

Pollan, B. (1993). *Samiske sjamaner: Religion og helbredelse*. Oslo: Gyldendal.

Pollan, B. (2002). *Noaidier: Historier om samiske sjamaner*. Oslo: De norske bokklubbene.

Turi, J. (1910/1965). *Mui'talus sámiid birra*. Stockholm: Skolöverstyrelsen.

Weber, M. (1971). *Makt og byråkrati: Essays om politikk og klasse, samfunnsforskning og verdier*. Oslo: Gyldendal.

World Health Organization. (2005). *National policy on traditional medicine and regulation of herbal medicines: Report of a WHO global survey*. World Health Organization.

World Health Organization. Retrieved from http://www.who.int/governance/eb/who_constitution_en.pdf?ua=1 (accessed on February 24, 2015).

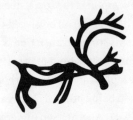

4

Dynamics of Naming
Examples from Porsanger

BARBARA HELEN MILLER

My research among the Coastal Sámi of Porsanger municipality spans
some 15 years. I was fortunate to have conducted many interviews with a
Coastal Sámi healer, Nanna, who lived from 1909 to 2002. In this chapter the
dynamics of naming is presented, and the examples I give will be from my
interviews with Nanna, her family, and her patients.

Naming is an idiom in the Coastal Sámi discourse on health and healing.
When I consider the local expressions of this idiom, my anthropological
view understands cultural knowledge as being socially distributed, in both
time and space, rather than found as a fixed stock of timeless and fully
shared models (see Shore, 1996, p. 260). There is a social life transforming
local terms, so a term may shift in its usage over time. Local expressions
of cultural models include many variations on the cultural model, and the
setting can be a factor determining the scope of the knowledge shared. An
example of the social distribution of Coastal Sámi knowledge is the healer's

knowledge that will not be distributed (or only partially or in a special setting) to his or her patients and family.

Correction, which for Nanna is "naming," is a tenet in the Sámi world view. However, endeavouring to determine the tenet exemplifies the social distribution of such knowledge. The tenet is basically that a spell can be placed—it is called *bijat* in Sámi and *gand* in Norwegian—but this simple translation is not straightforward. *Gand* is also used within the Sámi language but may carry a different interpretation than that of *bijat*. For example, a son of Nanna thought that one may never do *bijat*, but one may *gand* when being pressed or threatened. Nor is there agreement in the definition of *bijat*. Another son understood that *bijat* is used as a correction; this is close to Nanna's understanding, but her patients found that *bijat* was only "putting on the bad."

Observations of local practice include those of anthropologist Robert Paine. Paine did extended fieldwork in the 1950s on a Coastal Sámi village (south of Hammerfest) in western Finnmark. He uses the term *wizard* (indicating that in Sámi *noaidi* is employed) for the local practitioner and notes that the most common occasion for a wizard to use his power is to abort theft; a wizard is able to render a thief immobile until the wizard releases him. On other occasions a wizard is consulted to put a curse on someone who is felt to have caused an injury, and sometimes to remove such a curse (Paine, 1994, pp. 356-357). The placing of a curse or a spell (to immobilize) to which Paine refers is commonly called *ganding* in both Sámi and Norwegian. Social scientist Jens-Ivar Nergård (1994) considers that the sending of *gand* is a potential tool for justice within the community and that the Norwegian understanding of *gand* as sorcery is not correct. In the Sámi society, *ganding* is part of a justice system. When the *gand* can be lifted, it is judged to have been unjust, and this judgment will "hit" the one who had placed the *gand*. It means a loss of power for the *gander* (Nergård, 1994, pp. 137-142). For Nanna, the *gand* or the *bijat* is a correction, but she does not employ either term; she speaks of *naming*.

So we may ask, what does naming do? I posit the following for the dynamics of naming amongst the Coastal Sámi:

- The name forms a connection.
- There are right and wrong names. Right names further life; wrong names, or the lack of correct names, disrupt life.
- Naming is powerful, and an incorrect naming can come back to you.

- The right name is a part of the social relationships that build a complete person in a social environment.
- The name is established by baptism, and the connection is formed to the community, ancestors, and God.

I will give five stories, told to me during interviews,[1] which exemplify these dynamics. After each example the notions that inform this aspect of naming are elaborated, as clarified by either the interviewee or a family member or by examples collected during earlier interviews. The dynamics include a certain start-and-stop movement, and there are encounters that provide the logic for one thing happening over another.

The Fishing Boat

A family bought a new fishing boat. On its maiden voyage there was an accident. The next time they were on the sea, an accident happened again. Upon returning and relating these events the sons were told by their mother, "Give the boat a new name; the name is wrong" (*Bija ođđa nama, dán namma lea boastut*).

I have asked about the importance of a new name in this case (Miller, 2007, p. 93). One answer I received was that a name is associated with either good memories or bad memories, and changing the name makes it possible for the boat to be associated with good memories. This was also my interviewee's understanding of naming a child after the father and the grandfather, that is, the ongoing association of good memories with the name. The good memories carried by a name are considered to have value and must not be forgotten.

A family member of the interviewee said he would have expected that the change of name would have been the solution after a series of accidents, not immediately after the second accident. After some accidents it would be considered that the boat possibly carried a wrong name. He explained: "A name has a meaning. It must be a right name. If the name does not fit, it should be changed." He additionally explained that a name puts one on a path, and it can lead or connect in the right way or, if it is incorrect, in the wrong way. The understanding that a name has a meaning, and a changed name sets one on a new path, is also in the Bible, he said. The example is Simon, whom Jesus calls Peter, which means "rock." In Matthew 16, Jesus speaks to Simon: "Blessed art thou, Simon...thou art Peter, and upon this rock I will build my church."

The Grandchild

An elderly man in Lakselv related that he thought his grandchild had not been baptized as soon as the child should have been. His son and daughter-in-law had waited for a few months before the baptism. He felt that the delay had been unfortunate because the child had been crying during these months. He said that, as soon as the child received its name, it was quiet and content. (Miller, 2007, p. 93)

Delaying a child's baptism is considered unfortunate. There is a similar consideration when a child has been born who is not expected to live; haste is made to immediately baptize the child. Local hospital personnel will be familiar with this sense of urgency and keep the hospital chapel ready for an immediate baptism of the newborn in such situations.

The consideration in this example includes the understanding that for a child to be well it needs to receive a name, and that it is healthy when life is peaceful. Disruptions and accidents are indications of possible incomplete or incorrect connections, as was indicated in the renaming of the boat. These considerations are most clearly seen in the expectations for an unnamed newborn child who was left to die in an out-of-the-way place. Dead, the child is called an *eahpáraš* in Sámi. The *eahpáraš* haunts the location of its death; it has no peace. The *eahpáraš*'s complaints are heard when people pass close to the location. The solution to this disruption is provided by a healer, who will go to the location, talk to the *eahpáraš*, saying that it is now known what has happened, and the connection to God will be made, thereby lifting the haunting and putting the *eahpáraš* to rest (Miller, 2007, pp. 88–91).

The possible "spirit" of a location, or "presence" at a location, is at other times understood in terms of *gufihttarat* (subterraneous beings, in Sámi). A resident of Sandvik expressed her doubt that *gufihttarat* actually existed but nonetheless provided an interesting explanation for their existence: "I do not believe in these *gufihttarat*, but it is said that these are Eve's hidden children that she did not manage to wash before God came" (ibid., p. 83). Of note here is the notion that a water ceremony would be instrumental in establishing a complete social identity.

The activity of naming includes making corrections. The consequences of naming and correction are ingredients in the following example, which was told by Nanna. It involves a conversation between two healers, in which the definition of one given by the other is incorrect, and the enterprise backfires.

Competition

A local healer visited another healer because the local healer was not satisfied with what had been given and was interested in getting more. With this in mind, the local healer visited the other healer and tried to correct him. He answered, "Well, if you talk like a child, you will stay like a child." After this, she [the local healer] lost a lot.

What had initially been given to the local healer was her capacity to heal, which she had inherited from a former healer. We see in this story that she lost what she had originally been given. The intention had been to name (correct) the other healer, but it backfired when *she* was named (corrected) instead. The local healer in this case is understood by Nanna to be "corrected" by the other healer. Nanna considered the other healer to be correct in his definition of the local healer, because Nanna said that the local healer "after her visit became quite nervous," in other words, "will stay like a child." The other healer gave her a definition of herself that stuck. For Nanna there is a decisive moment in which the one being named does not have a choice; she employs the term *baptized* for this moment, and it is understood that one must accept the name (correction) or die. This understanding is even more clearly represented in the following story, but first we elucidate the local use of *baptized*.

The Sámi word for "baptism" is *gásttašit* and refers to a home baptism as well as a church baptism. The specific Sámi word for "a church baptism" is *risttašit*. There are more meanings for *gásttašit* than for *risttašit*; *risttašit* is only a church baptism. *Gásttašit* carries the meaning of "naming, correcting, and teaching." Additionally, in a game of cards *gásttašit* is the trump card. *Gásttašit* as "naming" is forceful and determining. It is interesting to note the root of the term, which is "to get wet." Also it can be noted from Håkan Rydving's (1993) study of religious change among the Lule Sámi that a water-pouring ritual was part of giving the name in pre-Christian practice; if a new name was needed, water was used to wash off the old name (pp. 115–117).

   Gásttašit's rich connotations are exemplified in the next example. It involves a healer, Johan Kaaven, who lived from 1836 to 1918 and lived close to where Nanna grew up.

The Neighbour's Daughter

Kaaven had requested from a neighbour that the man's daughter should come and work in Kaaven's home. The neighbour had answered, "Please don't request this. My daughter is needed in her own home." Kaaven continued to press his request and, after several attempts, placed a curse on the father's boat. The father, who was having troubles with his boat, consulted a man in Lyngen who was reputed to have special powers. The man from Lyngen said, "You have brought with you something belonging to Kaaven." Then the father was told that he would presently see how this would be returned. Kaaven met a whale. He was out fishing when a whale threatened to capsize his boat. He promised then and there to do the right thing, and the whale left.

This story is known locally because it appeared in Bergh and Edvardsen's (1990) book *The Man Who Stopped the Hurtigruta*, a collection of stories about Kaaven. However, Nanna had heard it from her parents. She said, "Kaaven confided to my parents that his work had caught him and corrected him" (*Kaaven dovddahii vahnemiidda ahte su dagut ledje juksan su, ja buorádahttán su*). Following closely the Sámi language in this statement, we can call attention to the ways in which a healer may be referred to. Nanna says *juksan*, and this is understood as "what was returned." The Sámi term *juovssaheaddji* is "one who returns," and it is one name employed for a healer.

Additionally we can note the Sámi word *buorádahttán* for "correction." *Buorideaddji* more closely translates as "improver." The root *buorre* means "good," and *buorideaddji* is also one of the ways to refer to a healer in Sámi.

Another comment made in Sámi by Nanna regarding this incident was, "The Lyngen man baptized Kaaven" (*Ivgoáddjá gásttaši Kaavena*). She continued, "Kaaven saw that he had no choice for 'who' he was going to be, if he would continue to live. Kaaven understood that his intrigue was sent back, he was about to be caught, and he promised conversion" (*ja son dagai buorádusa*). In the Christian context, conversion radically changes identity; one becomes born again in Christ. My interviewees were Christian or Laestadian, and their understanding of conversion implied this Christian context. However, it is significant that conversion also expresses Nanna's understanding of "correction" and "improvement."

The Rude Man, as Related by Nanna

Once a couple visited for my help, and I treated the woman. She said to her husband that they should pay. The man said that he did not think it was necessary to pay for this treatment. He seemed to think he had spirit powers. He was rude, and the couple left without paying. Within an hour the woman came back. She told me that her husband had collapsed while walking up the second hill, and asked if I would come. No, I would not come, and said to get an ambulance. But the woman kept asking, and finally I said, "Here is a glass of water from me. Tell him to drink it." The woman said that he would not drink it. I said, "Yes, he will." Indeed he did drink the water and could move on. Later he came and apologized for his rudeness.

The collapse of the rude man is a momentary paralysis, which can be a motif in stories where a healer has been wronged; it can also be the immobilization used to stop a thief. The dynamics of naming that we are observing, in correction and baptism, are contained in this story. We can look closely at what Nanna said in her statement about the man, and find her view. She said, "The man seemed to think he had spirit powers." In this statement Nanna indicates that there was a challenge in the man's behaviour toward Nanna, a challenge of "who can define whom." When the man left, he attempted a definition of Nanna; he identified her as someone who was "of little value." He named her. If this name for Nanna ("of little value") had stuck to her, he would be the one who could correct. However, the name was not correct, and therefore it did not stick to Nanna. One option for Nanna would have been to simply shrug off the name, but what this story tells is that Nanna used her other option, her capacity to name him correctly. Nanna said, when referring to this incident, "He was baptized." She did not say, "I baptized him." The correction is a process, and the person involved chooses whether or not to accept the teaching. The acceptance of the teaching was also considered to be the important element in Kaaven's encounter with the whale. Nanna employs the term *baptized* for this special, decisive moment, in which the person being named has no other possible choice for his or her identity; the person is baptized.

Considering the Practice of Renaming

Qvigstad (1932, p. 10) recorded that the Sámi concept of renaming was, in some cases, the understanding that the new name eluded the sickness demon. Rydving (1993) shows that the clergy during the seventeenth century considered the Lule Sámi to be Christian because the naming, marriage, and burial were largely performed according to Christian observances. However, unbeknownst to the clergy, the Sámi rituals for naming continued. After returning home from a Christian baptism, the child had the Scandinavian name washed off and obtained its Sámi name through a water-pouring ritual; additionally, the child received a certain theriomorphic guardian spirit, a *nimme-guelie* (name-fish) (Rydving, 1993 pp. 115–116). Rydving's sources on the north Sámi emphasize that children became ill and started to cry after the Christian ceremony, and therefore there was an urgency to receive a new Sámi name (p. 117). We are reminded of our story earlier in which the elderly man did not want to delay the baptism (or naming) of his grandchild, seeing that the child was crying; the child stopped crying after being baptized.

Rydving (1993) shows that during preceding centuries "one's name was an aspect of identity for the [Lule] Saami. To every name a certain identity was tied, to every identity a name" (p. 127). Today the local idiom of naming continues to indicate the understanding that to every name a certain identity is tied. Rydving states, "I do not interpret the Saami naming customs in 'soul'-terms" (p. 117n 94). I support Rydving in his choice not to interpret the naming customs in soul-terms, in particular because the use of the word *soul* can obscure, more than reveal, the local idiom. I find this to be the case in Pentikäinen's (1984) assessment of the healing ritual that he observed, in which his interpretation includes "robust soul." He writes, "The patient acquired a new, more powerful name and thus a new, more robust soul" (p. 128). Pentikäinen's identification of name and soul is not supported by ethnographic data; what the local healer or patient actually said is not presented. Moreover, instances of providing a new soul, as part of a healing process, are not found in the available data.

Locally the term *soul* is used only in its Christian context and understanding. For example, my interviewee said, "We all have an immortal soul." Significantly, the word *soul* during the religious change, that of Christianizing, did not receive an equivalent existing Sámi word; the Sámi language uses *siellu*, which is the Sámi's use of the Norwegian *sjel* (soul). *Spirit* is given many applications within the Sámi language. The Sámi whom I interviewed did not conflate spirit and soul. The recognition of the importance of the distinction between soul and spirit concerns the regional understanding of the location of the activity being described. Soul, for those Sámi interviewed, has a location in man himself and is personal—"my immortal soul"—even as a man's soul may go to the Christian heaven after his death. Spirit is not necessarily in man or otherwise connected to him personally; spirit is located outside, and a connection can be formed. An important regional consideration for health is the connection to or relationship with what is considered to be spiritual.[2]

The word *robust* obscures another clear distinction made in Sámi language usage. The Sámi terms *luondu* and *meahcci* have no exact equivalents in Norwegian, and both receive the translation *natur* (nature). *Luondu* is understood to speak of the human nature, the nature of an animal, the nature of the landscape, or the nature of the sea, etc. *Meahcci* is about resources in nature, the material for sustenance, such as the place for gathering berries or fuel. With the change in the economy, it became also a place in nature used for leisure. Activities on the land are called *meahcásteapmi*. However, it is interesting to note that, for example, when cows are brought to a grazing place in nature, they are said to go into *luohtu*. Important for the present discussion is *luonddohuvvat*, which translates directly as "I lost my nature," but the understood meaning is "I lost my energy." Therefore stating *robust*, and suggesting that renaming is the replenishing of energy, is not the indication. Additionally, *baptized* is used locally like a trump card, for example, in a convincing political debate in which there is no other choice and one is forced to accept the other opinion. The working of the trump card is not that the person's nature has been changed, but rather that the trump card establishes the path of evaluation. So again, a notion of "changing the nature" is not indicated by renaming. The name puts one on a path. When there are accidents and illnesses on this path, then the name is "wrong," and a new name should be given. The name gives direction, be it in action or in thoughts, which is (again) what being connected to an identity does.

Water and Naming

The aetiology for the Sámi term *gásttašit* (baptism) is "making wet." The use of water has been mentioned in many of the naming rituals so far, even in the case of Nanna and the rude man: Nanna offered him a glass of water. What is water within Sámi culture? It can separate or wash off unwanted connections, and it can make the correct connections, as water does in establishing the correct name during baptism. In the examples of water's use, we note the earlier-mentioned story, explaining the origins of the subterraneous beings, called *gufihttarat*. These beings were said to be Eve's children whom she did not manage to wash before God arrived. Not being washed, they lack a complete human social identity. Their relationship to God and ancestors is incomplete. They lack the connection, as was also the case for the *eahpáraš*. The connection to God had not been established, and therefore the *eahpáraš* stayed at the place of its death, rather than being able (if it had had a name) to join God and ancestors in heaven. To further explore and exhibit water's use for separating unwanted connections, we can refer to the accounts of Kaaven's healing practice (the healer who was threatened by the whale). One practice employed by Kaaven was to have a patient stand in the Porsanger fjord on a large rock during low tide, wait until high tide, and then walk through water to the shore. The notion was that the patient's illness would be separated from him; the illness could not stay attached to the patient going through water. This is similar to Qvigstad's (1932) report cited earlier that the renaming was thought to elude the sickness demon.

The name has a spiritual connection. Just what that connection is, is known by the successful healer. This was demonstrated in the story of the unsuccessful healer's trying to name another healer, and in the story of the rude man's unsuccessful attempt to name Nanna. I understood a cautionary instruction from Nanna to be "You ask spirits you know," because an unknown spiritual connection could be connected to something "bad." Incorrect behaviour that receives attention from a healer can result in a momentary paralysis for the one exhibiting it. This may be interpreted locally as a spell being placed by the successful healer, but the healer may see the momentary paralysis as simply the returning of the "bad" that had been unsuccessfully recruited by the now afflicted one. The rude man attempted to gain spiritual assistance. His attempted recruitment is expressed by Nanna, as follows: "He seemed to think he had spirit powers." The returning of the "bad" was also demonstrated in the story of Kaaven: the "bad" put on the fisherman's boat by Kaaven returned in the form of the threatening whale. For Nanna, the incident meant that Kaaven was baptized and that he needed to accept the correction or teaching, or die.

I hope to have shown that the cultural script of health amongst the Coastal Sámi of Porsanger includes the correct name. The name is a means for making connections, and the correct connections are healthful. When all is well, there is peace. Accidents, agitation, and unrest raise questions about correct connections. Then, as the above examples demonstrate, experiencing correction can be unsettling, to say the least. But when the teaching is accepted, there is again peace. The correct name has been established.

Notes

1. See Miller (2007).
2. Based on these arguments I am at odds with Hultkrantz's formulation in terms of "free-soul" for earlier Sámi shamanic practice (as in Hultkrantz, 1962–1963, p. 335).

References

Bergh, R., & Edvardsen, E.H. (1990). *Mannensom stoppet Hurtigruta: Historier og sagn on noaiden Johan Kaaven.* Oslo: Gøndahl & Søn Forlag.

Hultkrantz, Å. (1962-1963). The healing methods of the Lapps. *Arv, 18-19,* 325-351.

Miller, B.H. (2007). *Connecting and correcting: A case study of Sámi healers in Porsanger.* Leiden, Netherlands: CNWS.

Nergård, J.I. (1994). *Det skjulte Nord-Norge.* Oslo: Ad Notam Gyldendal.

Paine, R. (1994). Night village and the coming of men of the word: The supernatural as source of meaning among Coastal Sámi. *Journal of American folklore, 107,* 343-363.

Pentikäinen, J. (1984). The Sami shaman: Mediator between man and universe. In M. Hoppál (Ed.), *Shamanism in Eurasia,* part 1 (pp. 125-147). Göttingen: Herodot Forum 5.

Qvigstad, J. (1932). *Lappische Heilkunde.* Oslo: Instituttet for Sammenlignende Kulturforskning, Aschehoug & Co.

Rydving, H. (1993). *The end of drum-time: Religious change among the Lule Saami, 1670s-1740s.* Uppsala: Acta Universitatis Upsalienas, Historia Religionum 12.

Shore, B. (1996). *Culture in mind: Cognition, culture, and the problem of meaning.* Oxford: Oxford University Press.

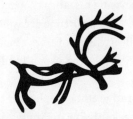

5

Multiple Views from Finnmark

KJELL BIRKELY ANDERSEN, SIGVALD PERSEN,
AND BARBARA HELEN MILLER

Idioms of Sámi health and healing convey the culture's interpretative tradition, the significance given to events that comprise social reality (Ramirez
& Hammack, 2014). The narrative in its construction makes meaning of the
social environs and, in so doing, employs local idioms. Engagement (by the
psychotherapist, traditional healer, or community) with an individual's life
story can be therapeutic, helping people to understand their experience
and construct a valued identity (Kirmayer, Dandeneau, Marshall, Phillips,
& Williamson, 2011), which can ensure vitality and a sense of agency; as
such, it leads to resilience that is interactive and contextual. Thus resilience
is available for an individual when there is "enough" engagement with the
multiple discourses composing their life world. Health seekers are challenged to engage with multiple discourses in post-colonial environments,
having been subject to extensive assimilation policies.

In the present chapter we attempt to show the state of the art, so to
speak, of the engagement with multiple discourses, placing side by side

the experiences of a local psychotherapist, a help seeker, and a traditional healer. We can observe (1) how the psychotherapist develops an understanding of his Sámi patient's coping strategies; (2) the patient's search for understanding; and (3) the traditional healer's basing his efficacy on participation. We observe how Sámi idioms for health and misfortune are woven into the local life experience. One idiom that effectively expresses a lack of vitality and the absence of agency is, in Sámi, *bijat* (placing a spell), and, in Norwegian, *gane*.

The methodology for this chapter is collaborative ethnography. The three authors present the health narrative of a help seeker living in Finnmark. We use the convention of the last name for the author and a first-name pseudonym, Hildegard, for the narrator, and personal identifying features have been left out. Hildegard has reviewed our use of her narrative and generously given her permission. Andersen gives a detailed account of his psychotherapeutic development, acquainting us with the environment encountered by Hildegard that includes multiple misunderstandings by health professionals. Persen provides the context and perspective of the one who has been consulted for his help. Miller recorded Hildegard's health narrative (presented in this chapter after Andersen's exposé) and provides concluding remarks.

Kjell Birkely Andersen

Hildegard's health narrative bespeaks her experience with modern medical practitioners; she was over-medicated, and their attitude was dismissive upon hearing of her use of traditional healing. My work environment is psychiatry, and as a local psychotherapist I can help to contextualize Hildegard's experience.

I have been working as a psychotherapist in the health-care system for some 15 years. My education is within the modern medical model, including studies at University College Tromsø and a master's degree from University College in Hedmark (Andersen, 2007). Currently I am working at the Sámi Competence Centre for Psychiatric Health Care (SANKS, Samisk nasjonalt kometansesenter—psykisk helsevern). SANKS functions for all of mid-Finnmark and is responsible on the national level for the development of health care for Sámi people. It has three departments, one for adults in Lakselv, one for children and youth in Karasok, and one for research and development. The Sámi health component addressed by SANKS is that of epidemiology. The Sámi individual's health issue is defined using the modern medical model and then considered in terms of its prevalence and possible social component. Sámi within SANKS does not address health as defined by a Sámi world view. Also lacking in the psychiatric approach to Sámi individuals is a cultural profile interview, which I have recently understood to be already standard practice in psychiatry in multicultural environments such as Canada (see Kirmayer, 2012).

In the course of our usual work at SANKS we employ cognitive behavioural therapy, the reflecting process therapy developed by Tom Andersen and Jaako Seikula, dynamic psychotherapy, and medication. Exploring the Sámi individual's use and competence in self-healing or folk medicine is not a focus. My concern for inclusion of elements of Sámi life experience in our treatment program led me to do research early in my profession. For my master's thesis I focused on Coastal Sámi recovery and coping processes. In 2007 I did research in the Porsanger area, interviewing residents concerning a wide variety of Sámi idioms for well-being (Andersen, 2010). There are four research results mentioned here.

1. Residents found that going out in nature was health promoting.
2. They also found that it was health promoting to have a talk with someone with whom they had a trusting relationship. These trusted people were for the most part healers. I was surprised to learn that the majority of those interviewed did not consult a healer for a physical illness.
3. The Laestadian congregation considered it to be health promoting when "we are giving good thoughts to each other"; this was done also in prayers.
4. One fisherman told me that he had a dream that felt like a nightmare. This was during a five-year psychosis. His turning point came with his decision to explore the dream. He found the truth of his dream just outside his own doorstep; indeed the resources of fish and game were being stolen. His work with the dream gave him power rather than illness.

In addition to Sámi idioms for wellness, there are Sámi folk beliefs for illness; one is the understanding of *gand*. A basic local understanding of a *gand* is that a spell has been placed. For my psychotherapist colleagues and the psychiatrists working at the Centre there is no systematic employment of the patient's understanding of what we could call, in the case of a *gand*, Sámi idioms of distress. Looking at my own practice from the first years to the present time, I notice a change in my integration of Sámi idioms for well-being and distress, and I would like to present it in the following; it amplifies Hildegard's experience.

My initial work can be demonstrated by the cases of three brothers whom I treated during my first years of practice. These brothers had lost their reindeer herd in the 1980s, and in the subsequent years they had problems with alcohol and depression. I saw my work with them as directed toward their alcoholism and depression and used the diagnostics and methodology from my education in the "Norwegian system." The brothers each spoke to me about their worries that a *gand* had been placed on their family and that this could explain how they had lost their reindeer and why they continued to have such bad luck in their enterprises. At that time I did not include in my work with them their explanation of a possible *gand*; I thought, "It is not my job." The change I note in my present way of working is that now I will speak with the patient about their understanding of a *gand*, and as a possible recovery solution I might even suggest to them that they consult a traditional helper.

An example of the inclusion of Sámi idioms in my work at the present time is the case of an elderly man who recently consulted me. He had a great deal of pain around his heart. I asked him if he had had such pain before. He had had a similar pain during the 1960s. I asked him what he had done for the pain at that time. He told that there was a "big healer," Løvlund, during the 1950s and 1960s in Tana and that he had consulted Løvlund. I asked what the healer had done. He said, "Løvlund read some verses in the Bible." The patient also had a recent dream that reminded him of the healing experience he had had with Løvlund; the dream was, "My pain is gone—now only a small point." I suggested that he think about what Løvlund had said and to consider his dream. This was a way to encourage the patient to repeat what had helped him then. Later he reported that this way of thinking (repeating Løvlund's advice) had indeed helped him.

Another recent patient was a woman who was unable to go to work and had difficulties sleeping. During our sessions I heard that her son had died in an automobile accident, and in her youth a family member had been shot and killed. I also heard that previously she had experienced help from someone she defined as "more Laestadian." I asked her if it was possible to search out this helper. She did so, and later I heard that they had talked in a way that facilitated a process and that she had returned to work and was able to sleep.

These examples of inclusion of Sámi idioms for suffering and healing show a development because, as stated, inclusion was not part of my work in the beginning. To give an accurate picture of psychotherapy in Finnmark, I should reiterate that inclusion of Sámi idioms is presently not common among my colleagues. In our team of professionals the openness of speaking together about Sámi idioms is quite determined by whom one is speaking with on the team. For example, one psychiatrist originally from the south of Norway does not take Sámi idioms into consideration, and one CBT therapist employs only the CBT framework. Should something of a Sámi idiom be mentioned, both give the comment, "I don't believe." Among those colleagues who give some attention to Sámi idioms, my rough assessment is that these people have grown up locally, as I have. Another difference in approach between my own and that of some psychiatrists is not one that is related to Sámi idioms; the difference rests in relying either on the pharmaceutical remedy or on psychotherapy. For context accuracy it should be noted that an ideal balance of medication and psychotherapy is disputed throughout Europe. My own conclusion is that in Norway the pharmaceutical solution has too great a dominance. Both a psychiatrist's too quick (in my opinion) use of medication and a lack of understanding of the local life can play a role in my hesitation to refer a patient to a psychiatrist. I may think long and hard before making a referral when my experience has been that the psychiatrist immediately prescribes antidepressants, for example. There are cases in which antidepressants only block the patient's feelings, and this use is unfortunate because what is blocked is also the needed process; a depressed period can be a process. Another incorrect use in prescribing medication occasionally comes from the general practitioner, when the physician prescribes medication for anxiety and depression before the patient comes to us, so medication is prescribed without a thorough enough diagnosis.

An example of a combination of over-medication and a lack of local context can be seen in the following case. Recently a middle-aged fisherman consulted me. He had a psychiatric history spanning 20 years, and his diagnosis was bipolar disorder and attention deficit hyperactivity disorder, for which he had been prescribed lithium, Ritalin, and neuroleptic medication. The medication, however, had been ineffectual for these last 20 years. He presented with sleeping problems and was further referred to me because the other therapists found him difficult and possibly suicidal. What I found to have been overlooked in his previous psychiatric evaluation was the consideration of the fisherman's life experience. For a sleeping disorder, in this case, one needs to include in the assessment the fisherman's often extensive work hours. During the fishing season a fisherman can have a chronic lack of sleep, sometimes lasting for days on end. In earlier times it would not have been uncommon for a fisherman to have hallucinations owing to lack of sleep. Additionally, a bipolar diagnosis in the case of this fisherman could also have had more to do with a cultural style of spending money that followed the intensive work period, than to do with bipolar disorder. Another consideration for depression can include the changes made during the 1990s to the official fishing regulations whereby some local fisherman lost their legal rights to fish.

My approach in working with him (and one that may be said to have had better success) was to ask, "What do you do to help yourself?" I saw him one month later, and he was doing well. He had been walking in the mountains and had decided to discontinue all medication. After we had spoken together for some time, he told me that his grandfather had been a healer and that he himself was a helper. He added, "No one has ever asked me about these things. With you I can speak." My sense was that he had opened up to me and that we had met on a totally different base than he had experienced with his other therapists and psychiatrists.

Considering my own training and education and those of my colleagues, it is possible to say that the psychologists and medical doctors working in Finnmark have not learned about the local folk medicine and the people's own way of seeking help, and their common attitude is dismissive. There are exceptions, of course. General practitioners and psychologists in Finnmark who have a Sámi background (as I do) have the life experience that does provide for a more open and listening approach when health problems are discussed. Additionally there have been physicians in Finnmark originally from the south of Norway who had attentiveness to the local understanding of health issues, albeit quite rare. When meeting people, I do see it as necessary to know their thinking about their own health solutions; their coping strategies, understood and encouraged, can be beneficial.

Life and Health Narrative

Hildegard's health narrative, recorded by Miller on September 17, 2011, took place at her home. English was the spoken language. Hildegard is in her early forties. Her first years were lived on the family farm, and from her seventh to sixteenth years she attended boarding school (*internat*), which was the norm for her village because it was quite some distance from the nearest school.

> HILDEGARD: I grew up on the farm. We were eight children. Father's side had been farmers, mother's side reindeer herders. I went to *internat* from seven years old. Mother brought me and she left; I was not home again until Christmas, then to leave again after Christmas. This happened over and over again. The *internat* was so different from at home; the children in my village did not fight, but here the children were fighting. I was a scared rabbit, always in a corner. I had a two-years-older sister, but she was embarrassed of me. Inside the *internat* we spoke Sámi and had Sámi teachers. I had difficulty in understanding the Norwegian teachers. We were left on our own; we did not have any help to dress. I could be seen as coming from a poor family because I did not have other shoes than Sámi footwear and homemade clothes.
>
> The school was for nine years. The hardest part was not to be with my parents, and during the last few years I was quite aggressive towards the teachers. When I was 16, I went back to my parents, living there for two years. My father had the idea that we needed to have a job; my feeling was, "Father, you don't want me home."

I went to work at the health centre, for old people, for two years. With the old people I recognized my own experience [at the boarding school] of being taken out of their home.

The boarding school experience was difficult, in particular because she was separated from her parents. She tried to find her way in further schooling but was not successful.

HILDEGARD: I went to Folk High School. By then I was not so afraid, a bit tougher. I had difficulties to concentrate on one thing, to study, so I took only a few courses. Then went to a school that was for three years, but I was too old [at 18] to finish it, so did only one and a half years, and studied English. Then back home at 19 years old and back to the Health Centre for a summer job. Then I went to school again, this time to Folk School for adults in the south of Norway. It was hard to be there; I had no entrance to the people. I got bad grades. There was a pressure from the family to get an education, but I only wanted to work. Then I moved back to Finnmark.

I was in Finnmark from my twenty-first to thirty-first years, and lived with a man for five years. I only had small jobs, perhaps because I was restless, I only could stay at a job for one or two years, and I travelled often. At a language school I taught Sámi for Norwegian speakers for two years. I was a grown-up woman and still had not chosen for an education; it was frustrating. My friends had studied. I did Sámi history and grammar at a high school—got bad grades.

Diligently overcoming obstacles, she discovered her real interest and found work successfully.

HILDEGARD: In 1998 I started a specialized training, and it felt right. I went to south Norway, just outside Oslo, and studied three modules. It was male dominated and even hard, but I loved it! To get into the training was difficult, but I received a recommendation from the civic defence, so I got in and finished in 2000. I took extra education and qualified. I immediately got work in Finnmark.

Hildegard encountered a problem in her boss and was not helped by her union:

HILDEGARD: I worked for eight years. And then I have been home on sick leave until the present. The problem has been my boss; I felt picked on. I realized that others got picked on—realized something was wrong with the boss. And told him, "You are not fair," and asked, "What have I done wrong?" Then things went really bad; he wanted me out of the way. He had already scared two people away. Our workplace had the highest percentage of sick leave; it is clear that others had the same pattern with this boss as I had. My decision has been to say, "This is not right." I contacted the union, and they have said, "We can't do anything" (the case for the last four years).

She was on sick leave and entered into a round of medical interventions:

HILDEGARD: I told my general practitioner that I thought I needed help, and he made the appointment with the psychologist. First I went every week and then after some months once every two weeks—in total one year. It did not help at all. I tried four different medications. I got sick to my stomach or a headache and was very tired. Most of the medication contained lactose, and I am lactose intolerant. The last medication was without lactose, but I was so tired, sleeping 12 to 15 hours a day. I told the psychologist, "I can't have this." He just listened and gave medicine. He suggested the Relax Centre in Tromsø. But I know who goes to this centre: they are those that need to leave home, their stress is at home; maybe they are beaten with an alcoholic husband. But I knew I wanted to be with my husband and to be in my garden. The psychologist despaired of me and said, "Now I don't know more." So after a year I ended this therapy.

However the NAV [Ny Arbeids og Velferdsordning (Work and Welfare Administration)] said, "You have to go for treatment for us to help you." But they have not helped—I have not received any financial support all these years. It is an unheard of situation. They say, "We cannot help, you have to quit your job." You see, all these years I am still employed. The employer offered a severance deal, to fix it and end the case. I refused. So to participate in this system I have to go back to another psychologist. I went to a psychiatrist, but they work with severe cases, and I am not sick enough. When we started, he believed me, he was calm. But this last summer he said, "Find a new job, get on with life." So then I saw he had not understood. I need to go for all possibilities.

Hildegard consulted traditional healers, also informing her general practitioner of this.

HILDEGARD: I heard that a woman from here had gone for cupping. I got his name and telephone number. I asked my mother and my sister to come with me. So in 2006 I went for the first time. At the first meeting I got cupped, I was a bit scared. I had headache, pain in my shoulders and back all the way to the tailbone. I got relaxed and slept well. He told, "So much stress and pain," and that I would have needed more cupping. Next time I went with my older sister and was again cupped, and, as the first time, I relaxed and slept well. The pain left for a few days, but this did not last; the pain returned. I went for a total of three cupping sessions. I had anxiety for cupping. I continue to talk with my healer about all my problems, mostly on the telephone.

In this period I went to two other Sámi healers. Already from childhood we went to healers; we went first to healers and only in the second place to modern medical doctors. My healer does a better job than the doctors here; that is, maybe doctors elsewhere, for example in Oslo, would have been good. The psychologist here did not understand me at all. At my place of residence I have seen three general practitioners. To the first doctor I said, "The only that has helped is healing. If I have fallen, for example, I go to the doctor only to register that I have these pains, for the system. But if I have bronchitis, then antibiotics work well." The doctor made no comment, but she put it in my file, as I found out during my visit to second doctor. He said, "I can see in your journal that you get healing. You cannot tell this to the doctor, because the doctor will think you are insane." I was shocked and without words. But then I said, "It is the most natural thing to talk about and to say." He said, "Doctors don't believe." I realized that he will never understand. The third doctor [many years later in 2010] was a young new doctor and asked what I had done for pain. I told him, "I'm coming to you as an alternative because my healer is so far away." He said, "You Sámi people still believe in that kind of shit in these enlightened times?"

She considered the working of traditional healing; there are possible spells (*bijat* in Sámi, *gane* in Norwegian) and God's power:

HILDEGARD: The healer can work for pains that have gathered in the body, for example through stress. Doctors give painkillers, but one reacts to medication, and this only makes it worse. And when there are troubles that the doctor cannot diagnose, he will say it is just hypochondria. The healers have their own specialities, and one does not know the speciality until you have tried them. And that is because what works for my friend may not work for me, and vice versa. Certainly by one healer I thought, "Never again." I found him stupid and thought this is not serious, all the talking and acting. One in Oslo started by praying to the four wind directions; this is not our tradition.

I have made the connection of Sámi healing with God, but now I think of nature itself and that a human can have this power. Laestadianism was important during my upbringing. In my area Laestadianism is very important. How that stays is in my respect for my mother; we children never argued with our parents.

I have asked healers about *bijat* and received different kinds of answers. One said, "No. No. Not possible. Don't even think—no one can *gane*." The second answered that they are not sure that someone is so bad and evil that they could cause pain and death. The third answered that, yes, they believe—it can happen. From my experience the healer does not like to talk about it. The stories I heard told from my area tell about the process. When there have been many unexplained problems, a person will go to one who can clean it up, take it away—there has been placed a spell. I understood cleaning it up used God's power. The one who put the spell uses dark energy, like sand from the graveyard. To take this away is used the power of religion, or one uses the same dark energy. My mother always said, "If you start to use these dark ways, they will control you." Even today I think, "All these things that have happened, [are my problems after all a *bijat*]?"

It is all around the world, in South America, "voodoo," they use these dark powers to do injury. A healer could lift the spell, and I would like to meet such a healer. But I imagine that only the older ones, those that are now dead, could do it. I don't know one, now, who I think could lift it. But I think, one has to put it somewhere, and so where? If on the road, innocent people might get it. And also one can never really know who put it—you cannot know. If accidents have been going on for 10 or 15 years, maybe the one who sent it would not know what he or she had done? It needs the confrontation, needs the "I am sorry," recognizing the wrong. Otherwise nothing is corrected; it is not solved. I am not sure if it is possible to put on a spell.

Sigvald Persen

My view is informed by my perspective of having been asked by local people for help. Hildegard's health narrative brings up several issues that are points of interest for people here: locating someone who might help, the course of treatment, and the expectations. I will additionally posit what I consider to be an important ingredient in this help, that of participation and the spiritual connection.

There are local expectations of help, and therefore to define the help we can simply call it *traditional help*. Within this tradition one never claims to have healed, and there is only an offer to help. Being unfamiliar with this tradition, you may then wonder how, without any outward display, I am actually found and consulted. Basically this happens by word of mouth. In a common path to consultation, a person has a problem and then he or she asks friends or family, "Who could help?" Possibly my name is mentioned, and my telephone number is given. When we are speaking together over the telephone, many things can happen; one option is that we decide that he or she will come to my home. With this visit there are again many options; one choice is to cup. Before, during, and after the cupping we talk together. It is usual that within a few days after the treatment I am called and told how it went and how they feel now. Depending on the problem, they may return for cupping, with an interval of three weeks or half a year. In those cases where the person lives too far to come to my home, an option is to talk on the telephone. This may happen on a regular basis, which varies from once a week to once in a half-year.

I learned cupping from my mother, Nanna, who was perhaps the last person in this area who continued to cup. Our understanding of the way in which health is promoted by cupping is that inflammation is reduced and the body's recovery is facilitated. The aim of cupping is not bloodletting but rather the removal of the inflammation. The correct positioning of the cups is essential. When I have determined where to place the cups, small incisions are made with a razor; the cups are applied and regularly removed and rinsed of the blood until the cups contain not blood but a somewhat clear liquid.

The local expectations include what may be called a religious element. My understanding is that the working of what may be called religious involves eliciting the patient's own healing capacities, which I consider to be participation. The patient and I experience being part of the process. We may experience this during or following a careful listening on my part. Even in small, seemingly unimportant exchanges it is there, for example when the patient gives me a gift. It happens regularly that I receive a gift, which could be reindeer meat, fish, or cloudberries. I see this gift as a way that the patient shows, "I am a part of this." For me, it is here that the distinction is made between this way of helping and the medical profession (although many more distinctions could be made). In the modern medical approach the patient is prescribed, for example, medication, but the patient is not asked to experience being part of the process. This applies also to the doctor; he is not asked to experience being part of the process.

Participation is again the key to understanding the practice that I and others refer to as binding and unbinding. I can say to the one calling me, "Let us bundle our thoughts." To give a more extensive example, I listen. The caller tells of his or her discomfort, pain, or fears. I say something whereby it is clear that I have heard. The caller says, "Yes, yes." So again, I am listening, the caller is telling, and we collect (bind) these thoughts that were, figuratively speaking, ghosting or haunting. The caller is then able to put these thoughts away. I am reminded of a helper who was active here during the first half of the twentieth century, Gamvik. My mother told that he solved a haunting (*eahpáraš*) by first listening and then saying, "Now we have heard the story."

There is certainly caution in traditional healing when defining. When I look back in time, it seems that this carefulness was found to be necessary. Within Laestadianism it seemed necessary to say, "We are dealing with something we know"; that is, "We know what spiritual connection this is." Therefore today the traditional helper is referred to as a "reader" and not a *noaidi*. This is necessary because at that time *noaidi* was understood to include a spiritual connection to both good and bad and, even further, to what one knew nothing about. It was understood that the *noaidi* used these connections as long as they supported his or her purpose, and this purpose was not always a good one. When I listen to my mother's explanations, I hear that people wanted to get rid of these bad sides and that this was achieved within Laestadianism.

Barbara Helen Miller

In Hildegard's narrative we note elements that correspond to Andersen's and Persen's descriptions of the local use of traditional healing, particularly in her ongoing trust that the healer understands her distress. Her experience with the modern medical profession exhibits the professional's lack of recognition of local folk medicine, as pointed out by Andersen. However, she was somewhat confrontational when speaking to her physicians on the theme of folk medicine. She acknowledged that she had developed a more aggressive stance during the years in boarding school. This stance is again exhibited in her conflict with her boss, a conflict that she refused to resolve in any way that absolved the boss of responsibility. We can ask if this is a typically Sámi problem. We assess that Hildegard's fighting stance against perceived injustice is not typical. However, Andersen and Persen see that the *internat* experience has had quite a negative effect on the emotional life and development of Sámi children and that this is carried over into adulthood. Persen finds the outcome of the *internat* experience to be a typical pervasive passivity.

Hildegard was initially cupped by the healer. She found it helpful in relieving her pains and for inducing a restful sleep, but she was not totally satisfied. Hildegard considered the possibility of a *gane*, and she questioned healers. She concluded that healers did not wish to discuss the question and that those who could have dealt with a *gane* were no longer living. Her approach to the question of a *gane* is quite typical of the Sámi population interviewed by Andersen and known by Persen, even though there are local differences. Persen has found the question of a *gane* to be relatively infrequent on the coast, when compared to inland populations of which Hildegard is a member. Her healer did not diagnose Hildegard's problems to be those of a *gane*. She was perhaps slightly disappointed in this and searched for other healers. Hildegard's understanding of a *gane* (the way it is expected to function) can help clarify her ongoing speculation. A *gane* can be instigated ritually, proceeding from a neighbour's anger and malice. The *gane* continues to bring ill fortune until it is either sent back or lifted or cleared by the expert. Persen's understanding that within Laestadianism it was found necessary to support only "known," and thereby "good," spiritual connections was not familiar to Hildegard. This is perhaps an example of local differences. The members of the local Laestadian congregation are, first of all, one's neighbours. Persen refers to the change that took place within his mother's lifetime whereby the local congregation managed to make a shift, deciding jointly to no longer make use of the "bad." Hildegard has some sense of the religious element that traditional helping might contain; however, she does not express a clear location of or connection to the religious element; she does not place it within the bounds of Laestadianism and only vaguely speculates that there is power in nature. She clearly recognizes the practice of the helping tradition, as seen in her narrative in which the practice of one whom she consulted was rejected as stupid, and another as "not our tradition." Persen's understanding of the religious element, that of participation, does not appear in Hildegard's narrative. Here Hildegard is not dissimilar to other help seekers who expect a religious element without having a clear concept of how or when the help works religiously; however, they do expect that clearing up a spell requires God's power. Persen's example of the clearing up of a haunting shows that witnessing confession ("Now we have heard the story") can be instrumental in restoring peace. Hildegard does share this notion for lifting a spell; she said, "It needs the confrontation, needs the 'I am sorry,' recognizing the wrong. Otherwise nothing is corrected; it is not solved."

The reason that Hildegard, in spite of her life experience and negative evaluation, consulted the modern medical practice for her complaints should be clarified. Her explanation—"So to participate in this system I have to go back to another psychologist"—means that the NAV (the Norwegian unemployment and welfare system with its protocol) stipulates that diagnostic and treatment advice has to be given by a modern medical practitioner in order for the patient to receive financial support.

Primitiveness and Participation

Andersen and Hildegard assessed critically some medical doctors and psychiatrists for their limited acceptance of the Sámi helping tradition. The general impression given by these professionals was that the Sámi helping tradition was primitive. We may understand such condemnation as a continuation of the late-nineteenth-century anthropological speculations characterizing so-called primitives in terms of a pre-logical mentality. Edward Burnett Tylor (1832–1917) saw religion as grounded in error (Lambek, 2002, p. 22). There was, however, an extensive anthropological debate (see Shore, 1996), a veritable cognitive revolution, during the mid-twentieth century that stripped this evolutionary framework of its validity (see Bloch, 1998). For some time Lévy-Bruhl was a central figure in this debate, and "participation mystic" was his influential idea (Lévy-Bruhl, 1910/1926).

Lévy-Bruhl's principle of participation is useful in modern anthropological research, but only when shorn of ties to cultural evolution so that "participation" does not describe the quality of mysticism attributed to *primitive* religious thought. Participation proposes correspondences or relationships where at other times the same group or individual would propose differences and oppositions. Collective representations legitimize mystical thinking, and each culture (present-day and past) has its representations whereby participation is made operational (see Shore, 1996, p. 28). Lévy-Bruhl's helpful characterization of participation shows that concepts are also sensuous, coloured by bodily activity, and therefore significant for the embodiment of human understanding.

Participation's significance for the embodiment of human understanding brings into focus the way in which a helping practice that engages with local idioms can be at an advantage over help that is not grounded in local knowledge. Certainly the communication between seeker and helper, between the illness and life experience, is optimized by cultural imagery. This emphasis can be found expressed by anthropologist Clifford Geertz. Commenting on culture theory, he stresses the human need for symbolic models of and for reality: *"the human brain is thoroughly dependent upon cultural resources for its very operation*; and those resources are, consequently, not adjuncts to, but constituents of mental activity" (Geertz, 1973, p. 76; italics in original). The same understanding is expressed in neuroscience. Neuroscience research can now explain how the brain has the capacity for neuronal reconfiguration; this is our brain's plasticity and capacity to recover. This plasticity becomes operational with imagination and works in relationship to cultural expressions (see Paris, 2011; Solms, 2002). Edward Said (1993), a founding figure in the critical-theory field of post-colonialism, has postulated that in spite of good intentions, expert and global knowledge systems have routinely undermined and overruled the local knowledge system, to the disadvantage of local populations (see Skovdal, 2012, p. 483).

Answers from Transcultural Psychiatry

The role of culture in mental health is importantly discussed in anthropological literature (Kirmayer, 2006; Kleinman, 1980). Laurence Kirmayer, psychiatrist and anthropologist, developed a model for accessing the patient's cultural perspective on wellness and illness called the "cultural consultation" (Kirmayer, Groleau, Guzder, Blake, & Jarvis, 2003). Arthur Kleinman, psychiatrist and professor of medical anthropology and cross-cultural psychiatry at Harvard University, argues for the recognition of the local distinctions, the cultural distinctiveness. He was instrumental in developing what was termed the "cultural formulation" for the publication of the new psychiatric diagnostic manual, *Diagnostic and Statistical Manual of Mental Disorders 4* (DSM-4, 2000), having co-chaired the American Psychiatric Association's Task Force on Culture and DSM-4. The addition of the question of culture to the DSM is new to its publication; DSM-3 (1980) did not contain clauses alerting psychiatry to the mediating factors of cultural diversity for diagnosis (see Swartz, 2012).

The relatively new field of transcultural psychiatry has criticized mainstream psychiatry for fostering a "one-size-fits-all" international diagnostic system for mental disorder. Transcultural psychiatry shows that mental disorder may manifest differently in different parts of the world, and (among other efforts) tries to understand so-called culture-bound syndromes. Its critical research in psychiatry contests the foundational assumption of Western psychiatry, which considers that mental disorder can be viewed with the use of quantitative methods based on Western models of symptomatology, without including the contexts of society and culture (Summerfield, 2012, p. 523). The research of transcultural psychiatry attests to the direct and indirect health-enhancing impacts of positive local participation in community activities, be they related to friendship or spiritual faith (Campbell & Burgess, 2012, p. 387).

Derek Summerfield (2012), psychiatrist and researcher in transcultural psychiatry, criticizes the overrepresentation of big pharmacy in psychiatric treatment plans and considers that people could be better helped by psychiatry's focus on understanding the way in which the patient copes. Summerfield considers that without assessing a whole person as he or she is immersed in the complexity of life, so-called mental illness can be misdiagnosed; the patient's symptoms may be rather normal reactions to negative circumstances (p. 520). Morten Skovdal (2012), community health psychologist, argues cogently that when the conceptual tools through which meaning is given to distress are in the hands of global mental health, the focus is (too often) on vulnerability rather than on resilience, thereby ignoring local strengths and coping strategies (pp. 483–484). Coping can include the use of those tools made available by the cultural wealth.

These points of criticism made by transcultural psychiatry of Western psychiatry (basically of the non-inclusion of the cultural formulation and the over-use of medication) are the same criticisms of local psychiatric practice posited by Andersen. Andersen focused on the patient's own coping strategies, asking his patient, "What do you do to help yourself?" Hildegard's experience with prescribed medication, psychiatry, and psychotherapy can be seen as examples of Andersen's criticism of his profession: medication is not prescribed carefully enough, and psychiatry and the psychotherapist are not adequately aware of local life, with the result that there are instances of misdiagnosis and missed chances for employing the local avenues for coping. Andersen, in his research and considerations of the life world of his patients, is coming to the same conclusions as those of transcultural psychiatry.

Transcultural psychiatry also has points of agreement with the traditional helper's understanding of this help. The repair that the Sámi helper hopes to facilitate is both individual and social. Summerfield criticizes the Western psychiatric canon for flaws in its fundamental assumptions, that the human individual is the basic unit of study, that the mind is located inside the body, and "what is 'social' is outside the body and outside the frame of reference" (2012, p. 527). We have seen that the correct attitude of the Sámi helper is emphasized as an important promoting element. The participation, which Persen finds essential for healing, is also given credit by Summerfield. He finds that social participation advances the sense of coherence and that positive social connectedness is central for mental health (Summerfield, 2012, pp. 527–528).

Hildegard's symptoms of stress, of overall pains, and of sleeplessness may be diagnosed in the psychiatric terms of depression—post-traumatic stress disorder—but may be diagnosed by traditional healing as symptoms of dysfunctional social relationships. When mental illness is a biological illness, medication would indeed be indicated, but healing social relationships has been the task of cultural practices. One of the avenues in the Sámi culture has been the Laestadian meeting, the place in which to ask one's neighbour for forgiveness.

References

Andersen, K.B. (2007). *Å berges, Erfaringer om bedringsprosesser ved alvorlige psykiske lidelser i sjøsamisk område* (Master's thesis in Mental Health Care). Hedmark, Norway: Høgskolen.

Andersen, K.B. (2010). Å berges—en studie av noen brukererfaringer fra et sjøsamisk område. In A. Silviken & V. Stordahl (Eds.), *Samisk psykisk helsevernnye—landskap, kjente steder og skjulte utfordringer*. Karsjok, Norway: Čálliid Lágádus.

Bloch, M.E.F. (1998). *How we think they think: Anthropological approaches to cognition, memory, and literacy*. Oxford: Westview Press.

Campbell, C., & Burgess, R. (2012). The role of communities in advancing the goals of the Movement for Global Mental Health. *Transcultural Psychiatry, 49*(3–4), 379–395.

Geertz, G. (1973). *The Interpretation of cultures.* New York: Basic Books.

Kirmayer, L.J. (2006). Beyond the "new cross-cultural psychiatry": Cultural biology, discursive psychology, and the ironies of globalization. *Transcultural Psychiatry, 43*(1), 126–144.

Kirmayer, L.J. (2012). Cultural competence and evidence-based practice in mental health: Epistemic communities and the politics of pluralism. *Social Science and Medicine, 75*(2), 249–256.

Kirmayer, L.J., Dandeneau, S., Marshall, E., Phillips, M.K., & Williamson, K.L. (2011). Rethinking resilience from indigenous perspectives. *Canadian Journal of Psychiatry, 56*(2), 84–91.

Kirmayer, L.J., Groleau, D., Guzder, J., Blake, C., & Jarvis, E. (2003). Cultural consultation: A model of mental health service for multicultural societies. *Canadian Journal of Psychiatry, 48*(2), 145–153.

Kleinman, A. (1980). *Patients and healers in the context of culture.* Berkeley: University of California Press.

Lambek, K. (2002). *A reader in the anthropology of religion.* Oxford: Blackwell.

Lévy-Bruhl, L. (1910/1926). *How natives think.* New York: Knopf.

Paris, Ginette. (2011). *Heartbreak: New approaches to healing.* Minneapolis, MN: Mill City Press.

Ramirez, L.C., & Hammack, P.L. (2014). Surviving colonization and the quest for healing: Narrative and resilience among California Indian tribal leaders. *Transcultural Psychiatry, 51*(1), 112–133.

Said, E. (1993). *Culture and imperialism.* London: Chatto.

Shore, B. (1996). *Culture in mind: Cognition, culture, and the problem of meaning.* Oxford: Oxford University Press.

Skovdal, M. (2012). Pathologising healthy children? A review of the literature exploring the mental health of HIV-affected children in sub-Saharan Africa. *Transcultural Psychiatry, 49*(3–4), 461–491.

Solms, M. (2002). *The brain and the inner world: An introduction to the neuroscience of subjective experience.* New York: Other Press.

Summerfield, D. (2012). Afterword: Against "global mental health." *Transcultural Psychiatry, 49*(3–4), 519–530.

Swartz, L. (2012). An unruly coming of age: The benefits of discomfort for global mental health. *Transcultural Psychiatry, 49*(3–4): 531–538.

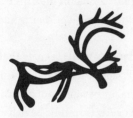

"Suffering in Body and Soul"
Lived Life and Experiences of Local Food Change in the Russian Arctic

TRINE KVITBERG

Now I have such a feeling of having it bad. We don't see reindeer meat anymore. No places to get it. It's only if you know someone, and only if they deliver meat to the military farm for an exorbitant price. I personally feel bad. I am suffering in body and soul!
(Anna, in Lovozero)

Introduction

Climate change and environmental pollution have become pressing concerns for the people in the Arctic region (Young, Rawat, Dalimann, Chatwood, & Bjerregaard, 2012). The health of indigenous women in the Arctic is affected by the global voyage of pollutants that enter the bodies of Arctic animals and then the bodies of women, girls, unborn generations, and Arctic indigenous peoples as a whole.[1] The consumption of local food in indigenous communities is highly relevant to health.

Some researchers link climate change and changes in living conditions to human health. A number of studies have provided data on the differentiating effects of climate change on women's and men's well-being and health (Kukarenko, 2011).

The Intergovernmental Panel on Climate Change (IPCC)[2] reports that women constitute up to 70 per cent of the world population that lives under the poverty level. Still, women and their personal experiences of health and illness are repeatedly absent both in global or Arctic public health research and in the IPCC document. Voices of elderly indigenous women are seldom heard.

Voices not heard, or the suppression of personal biographies, is conceptualized as "structural violence"[3] in critical medical anthropology (Das, 2007a; Farmer, 2004). Social inequalities are at the heart of structural violence (Farmer, 2004, p. 317). Structural violence is embodied as adverse events if what we study, as anthropologists, is the experience of people who live in poverty or are marginalized by racism, gender inequality, or a noxious mix of all of the above (ibid.). The adverse events discussed by Farmer include epidemic disease, violations of human rights, and genocide. Indigenous women are vulnerable to structural violence.

An objective of this present research is to add awareness to stories of Arctic elderly indigenous women and their health and illness experiences in the age of climate crisis. The stories focus on lived life and experiences of change in the local food in the Arctic. I draw attention to a critical medical anthropological perspective that contributes the concept of social suffering to public health studies. The experience of suffering brings into a single space an assemblage of human problems that have their origins and consequences in the devastating injuries that social forces have inflicted on human life. Social suffering results from the effects of political, economic, and institutional power on people (Kleinman, Das, & Lock, 1997). Das (2007a) emphasizes critical events and contributes to the thinking on violence and the way it affects everyday life. Instead of asking how we should look at the problem of violence, how we can logically grasp it, Das asks *who hears this voice* (Das, 1995, p. 162). When we listen sensitively and let stories happen to us, this will in turn affect the way we present our ethnography (ibid., p. 166).

The voices of elderly Russian Sámi women and their health and illness experiences are absent in Arctic public health research. The aim of this chapter is to show how sensitive listening to personal food biographies adds to the awareness of the health and illness experiences of elderly Sámi women in the Russian Arctic.

First I present the setting of this study, Lovozero on the Kola Peninsula, a brief description of the critical events of the Russian Sámi, and then some words about sensitive listening in ethnographic interviews. Thereafter the events of Anna's life are described primarily in her own voice. To conclude I draw out some of the events and analyze them from a critical medical anthropological perspective.

The Setting

Lovozero on the Kola Peninsula in northwest Russia was selected for ethnographic interviews of elderly indigenous women regarding their food consumption. The selection was made in a preliminary research protocol by the Arctic health research team at the University of Tromsø. Food and health security in the Kola region is an aspect of Arctic health research.

In the Russian Arctic the greatest sources of pollution are the oil and gas industries, as well as mineral extraction and processing, aggravated by poor purification facilities. One of the main negative impacts of industrial development that is threatening the livelihood of indigenous people, which is mentioned in the Arctic Climate Impact Assessment (ACIA) report, is the flooding of especially valuable subsistence areas in the construction of hydroelectric power dams (Nuttall, 2005, p. 678).

Lovozero is the present centre of Sámi settlement in the peninsula. The village is located 180 kilometres south-southeast of Murmansk. Kola Peninsula has nearly one million inhabitants, about half of which live in Murmansk. The dominant nationalities are Russian and Ukrainian. Lovozero has approximately 3,500 inhabitants and is the administrative centre for 15,000 inhabitants. The local inhabitants live in large apartment blocks in Lovozero and are Russians, Ukrainians, Komi, Nenets, and Sámi.[4] The three indigenous groups of Sámi, Komi, and Nenets have had a different status in relation to the Soviet authorities. They have also competed for the

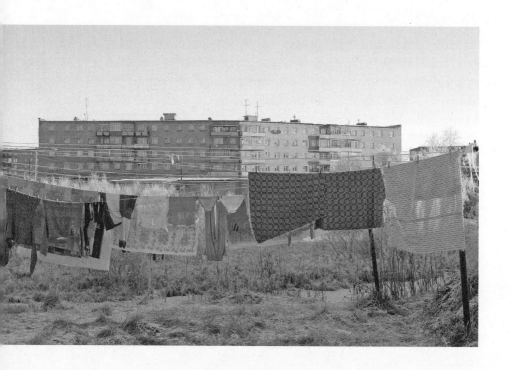

Laundry hanging out to dry between apartment blocks in Lovozero, Kola Peninsula, Russia. Photograph by Trine Kvitberg.

same resources. In Lovozero there are many elderly women living alone in small flats in the large apartment blocks.

Critical Events

Jelena Sergejeva (2000, p. 5) gives a short account of the history of the Russian Sámi or the Eastern Sámi (Inari, Skolt, Akkala, Kildin, and Ter Sámi) that I use in this section. The whole Sámi population was originally divided into social entities (*sijdds*) consisting of certain families and kin. At the beginning of the nineteenth century the *sijdd* system started to change under the influence of state politics and the economic development of the area. Gradually many Sámi families had already ceased to practise their semi-nomadic reindeer-herding way of life and had settled permanently in their traditional areas.

During the twentieth century the great majority of the Eastern Sámi were forced to leave their traditional areas of habitation. A breakdown of the Sámi identity started when the traditional Sámi way of life was suppressed. The crisis of the Sámi in the Soviet Union reached its peak during the 1950s and 1960s, when the remaining Sámi villages were razed to the ground and all the inhabitants were removed by force. Their economic structure and means of livelihood broke down completely. This major and critical event had a deep impact on the Russian Sámi's everyday life.

When the Sámi in the Soviet Union were displaced from their traditional dwelling places and moved to bigger villages, they lost their traditional way of life. Many families had to be accommodated in the homes of Lovozero (Luujaavv'r) residents, which resulted in overcrowding, and tensions were worsened by excessive drunkenness (Luk'jancenko, 1989, p. 130). The Sámi villages were characterized as "without perspective" (Mustonen & Mustonen, 2011).

In contrast to other Sámi in the West, the Eastern Sámi have been Orthodox Christians. However, over many decades Sámi in the Soviet Union, through the state's atheistic policy, were denied the chance of practising their religion.

Ethnographic Interviews

Through the help of ethnographic interviews, Veena Das (2007a) has shown how adverse life events for women are experienced as an inability to maintain domestic life. She shows the deep connection of the event and the everyday. In her book *Life and Words: Violence and the Descent into the Ordinary* (2007) she demonstrates the connection between gender and violence, and the way that violence can hide in the flow of ordinary everyday life. Das emphasizes that ordinary life requires work, and to think about the ordinary can be a kind of methodology. During very exceptional moments all kinds of everyday things have to continue to be done. She stresses that very often it is at this juncture that anthropologists lose interest in what is at stake. The kind of work that needs to be done to maintain the everyday, and the ways in which the ordinary and the extraordinary are braided together in our everyday lives, are, Das says, theoretically much more difficult to understand than the resistance model.

Veena Das emphasizes that there is a long history of thinking that ordinary life does not require work in order to be maintained, that it has the force of habit, and that therefore it goes on sustaining itself (DiFruscia, 2010, p. 137). These theories propose that methodologically one can best detect agency at moments of resistance because of the presumption that ordinary life just goes on. She says there is a certain kind of heroic model of resistance, a romance of resistance. Das's argument is to think about agency in much more complex ways. She calls attention to everyday life as a kind of *achievement*, not just as a part of habit.

Das, in her research, portrays personal biographies of women in Indian societies who had suffered the trauma of Partition, and she tells how they dealt with the poisonous knowledge of having witnessed unprecedented violence. She portrays one woman who was not herself subjected to violence, but the trauma of the violence transformed the world in which she lived. The events of the Partition became woven into the events of her life (Das, 1995, p. 167).

Sensitive Listening

Sensitive listening in ethnographic interviews can serve as a portal to a complex, embodied form of memory and perceptual experience. The senses are some of the strongest vessels of memory, and they work to provide a portal into experiences or stories that might otherwise remain untouched in a research situation (Harris & Guillemin, 2012, p. 693). Harris and Guillemin show, in an article about sensitive listening in qualitative interviews, how objects have been used as triggers for stories. The researcher can motion toward objects in a participant's living room, inviting the participant to speak about them and reflect on how he or she feels, opening points of memory. Sensitive listening is not restricted to a single sense. The senses are intertwined; once one is attuned to one sense, the other senses come to the fore (Harris & Guillemin, 2012; Ingold, 2000; Pink, 2009).

Sensitive listening means also not trying to define or explain, but only listening attentively to others. For the teller it is therapeutic. Anybody who carefully begins to express himself or herself steps into a healing process. It is healing when someone listens without interrupting, waiting for the other's words without an impatient attempt to fill the empty gaps.

A Story Waiting to Be Told

In autumn 2008, a Russian interpreter and I were invited to visit nine elderly Russian Sámi women and some Komi women in their homes in Lovozero. A few weeks earlier, during the Sámi summer festival, we had visited Lovozero to establish contact with the elderly Sámi women who would tell their food biographies.

Anna had a story waiting to be told. It is a story about the way in which ordinary Russian Sámi women have lived with major changes. Their everyday life was the hard and patient work required for that everyday life to be fulfilled. A major change in which Anna was deeply embedded was the displacement from her home village of Voronja on the Kola Peninsula. The event attaches itself with its tentacles into everyday life and folds itself into the recesses of the ordinary. It shows the slippery relation between the collective and the individual (Das, 2007a).

Audio Recordings

All field interviews were conducted in Russian with a Russian interpreter who translated into Norwegian. The interviews were also audio-recorded, and the transcription was made verbatim from Russian speech into Norwegian. Most of the interviews were transcribed and translated by my authorized Russian-Norwegian translator who was engaged in the field interviews. The last stage of translation from Norwegian to English was made by this author, the fieldworker. Field notes were recorded and used at several stages in the research process. The tapes were replayed, and the transcribed text was reread to allow us to experience Anna's story.

Anna's Story

Anna lives in a two-bedroom apartment on the fifth (top) floor of an apartment block in Lovozero (Luujaavv'r). When I came to Lovozero in November 2008, I was aware first of the silence. The roads were silent, the backyards were silent, and the stairways in the concrete blocks were all silent. In the stairways I could hear some voices from radios behind simple doors. The smell of old garbage that was piling up outside the blocks and in the stairways met us before we reached the fifth floor. Anna met us with a smile.

She opened the door and invited us into her apartment on this cold winter's day. Anna was wearing a beautiful headdress, and a colourful shawl covered her shoulders. With a handshake and a gesture of cordiality and hospitality we were welcomed into her apartment to the words "I have been waiting for you." Anna's friendly words and smiling eyes invited us in to listen to her story. Anna had prepared for the meeting. The table was set nicely with three cups for tea; a photograph album and a picture were placed in front of us. She had placed herself in the middle as though she were on a stage, and my translator and I were the audience around the table. Anna closed the curtains in the living room, and the grey apartment blocks outside were out of sight. The weak and very low Arctic sun shone through the curtains and into the living room. Anna started spontaneously to tell.

ANNA: Now I really want to tell. I was born in Voronja in September 1949 in a Sámi family. We were *real* Sámi. There were no mixed marriages. There was only Sámi blood. We were herding reindeer at home. We had reindeer and not just a few.

Anna repeated again and again that they were *real* Sámi. She told me to write it down in my notebook.

On the wall in Anna's living room hung some pictures. One picture was of the Virgin Mary and the Christ child, and another picture was of Lenin, founding father of Soviet communism. On the table in front of us was a picture of the Kola Sámi creation myth "Father Myandash, the Reindeer Man," with a Sámi girl embracing his neck.

The living room was nicely decorated with Sámi *duodji*, handcrafted reindeer skin. Anna touched the reindeer skin very gently and gave it to us to touch and smell. The touching and the smelling of the soft reindeer skin in her hand evoked memories, and Anna continued telling. She leaned forward in her chair and with suspense guided us into her story. Anna told how she was trained to rely on the reindeer that always brought her safely home.

Father Was Far Away

ANNA: Do you know...? Now I want to tell you...When my father travelled to the forest to cut trees...He got storage for the wood and went far away into the forest. He was absent for many days. We had trained reindeer. My mother put food in a reindeer sleigh, harnessed the reindeer, and I went all alone out onto the taiga. It was me alone travelling out there to him with food. The reindeer were trained to remember the route. I was only a child who went off alone with food for my father.

"Did you travel all alone?" we asked.

ANNA: Yes, I am going to tell you now! I was six to seven years old. We were trained by our parents to take care of animals and the housekeeping. In Voronja there was only me who could handle the reindeer and the dogs. We also had four dogs, and they all were trained.

Anna told about the reindeer that guided her over the tundra and taiga. The reindeer remembered the way, protected her, and guided her safely through the landscape. Father was far away, but the reindeer was present.

Being a Good Son

Anna's face was suddenly expressionless. A gleam in her eyes asked if we were following her story. We nodded as a sign of our acceptance to follow her story.

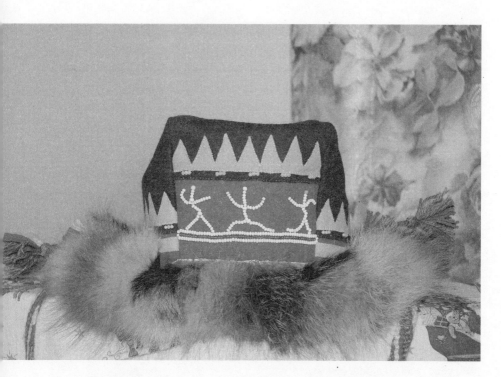

Kola Sámi *duodji* (handcrafted reindeer skin) arts and crafts. Photograph by
Trine Kvitberg.

ANNA: And I am going to tell you! My father started very early, from
five years old, to take me to his fishing places. He left me alone on an
island for a long time and did not allow me to be afraid. I was trained
not to be afraid of anything, not to show fear. When I was five years
old, I had to clean the fish and cook, keep the fire alive, and watch
the eye of the fish. I should remove the soul from the fish. When the
eyes of the fish came out, it was cooked. That was the sign. It was
terrible. I wept a little but had to do all the work. Then I took some
more firewood to keep the fire alive. When my father returned from
fishing—and my father was never alone; there were four who were
fishing together. They usually asked, "Why do you have red eyes?" I
said, "From the fire." I always said it was the smoke from the fire. I
never told I was crying. My father was waiting for boys. All the sons

died in childhood, but my father told me, *"Khoroshaya synok."*[5]
Do you understand?

Anna put intensity in her voice when she said *"Khoroshaya synok."* She told about a moment of intense emotion in her ordinary life.

Mother's Soup and Gifts of the Forest

We asked Anna if she could tell what she had eaten in the past. Anna remembered and spoke vividly and in detail about her mother, the food, and her home in the 1950s. Memories were evoked of the tasty and healthy soup.

> ANNA: My mother always said, "Everything in the soup is what humans need." Do you know how she was making the fish soup? This was the very best. She took different kinds of fish. She started with whitefish. She soaked, boiled the whitefish. In the same stock she put pike. Afterwards she soaked the pike and put perch in the same stock. It is considered the best fish soup. Then the children picked the green chives [*loafkhess*].[6] It tasted very delicious.

Anna's voice was lilting when she spoke about her mother and the memories of her mother's fish soup, *Kull lumm*,[7] from her childhood.

> ANNA: In Voronja it was so; there was always fresh milk, always reindeer milk and fresh cheese, and fresh sour cream, and reindeer butter. Everything was fresh. Everything was our own. When my parents went for the haymaking season…I am going to tell now; we prepared the berries. There were a lot of berries in barrels. It was cloudberries, cowberries, blueberries, whortleberries, crowberries. We picked crowberries, squeezed juice, and drank the juice. All winter we were drinking the juice of crowberries. Our parents froze the crowberries. We used the crowberries for fish soup. We ate flour soup. It could be flour soup with fish or meat [*Kull-vjarr*]. I remember that very well. My mother loved that soup.

Anna poured some more tea into our cups and continued her story in a lilting tone.

> ANNA: I remember my mother always gave thanks to the forest before she entered into the forest. When she went to the forest, she always said, "Thank you for the gifts of berries and mushrooms." And I do it too. I say honestly. I am still doing it. It's alive and it's breathing. I will always lean onto a lonely birch if it is alone. Certainly I will keep the palm of my hands to the sun and open my arms toward the sun. That's for sure. And do you know?

Anna looked at us. Her eyes were asking if we were following her story. She now raised her voice in a steady tone.

Major Changes in the Forest

> ANNA: But now we have no rights to visit the areas of the past. We have no rights to fish and pick berries. And it's *there* where it's the most berries and fish. We do not have any rights to fish there. No rights. It's no secret for anyone, but we are just fully banned. As soon as we are coming close to the shores, the fish inspectors pop up, and we are punished to pay, although nothing is caught.

"No access to the local food?" we asked. Anna raised her voice again.

> ANNA: And there have been major changes in the forest. Cry out that there are major changes now. When there are berries, we are harvesting. If not, it does not matter because the cloudberries are very poor. They are not getting mature. They are black at once. It's very few whortleberries and blueberries, very few. The most obvious sign of impoverishment is the rowanberries. It has been the most impoverished and dried up. The juiciness is lost. Potatoes are different now. In the past we were growing potatoes, but we stopped because of the high cost. We need fertilizer for growing, but it's too expensive to get. We buy the fertilizer at the state farm. Do you understand?

We listened with attention.

Suffering in Body and Soul

We asked, "How are your days?" Anna told us about her heart attack of several months ago. She spoke about the long and lonely days that she had spent in her chair, looking at her pictures. Anna showed us one of her beloved pictures, that of Father-Myandash, the Reindeer Man, with the Sámi girl embracing his neck. Anna told us how she had spent her days looking at this image and reflecting on her lived life.

I asked if she could tell us what she eats everyday. Anna's eyes answered with a question: "Do you accept my story? Do you want to hear? Do you follow me?" We responded by nodding, and I found some words in broken Russian to acknowledge that we were following her story.

> ANNA: Now I have such a feeling of having it bad. We don't see reindeer meat anymore. No places to get it. It's only if you know someone, and only if they deliver meat to the military farm for an exorbitant price. I personally feel bad. I am suffering in body and soul! Do you understand?
>
> When I eat reindeer meat! Oh, my God! My children are used to reindeer meat, my sons. Even if I only came with a little bit of reindeer meat, there was nothing left for making soup. We ate it raw.

Her face expressed a smile when she remembered the time of tasty reindeer meat.

> ANNA: Now...I tell you. Wintertime is slaughtering, and if we are lucky, we get half a carcass, but this is very rare. And we know by taste and smell it's not the same reindeer meat. The quality is changed. It is not juicy. It's dry, a dry meat.

Anna showed her hands and the dryness in her body. The skinfolds on her hands expressed dryness and the high weight loss that she had experienced after the heart attack. Anna spoke about the weight losses she had experienced in her life. She remembered how she lost weight and felt like drying up in those times when she did not see reindeer or have juicy reindeer meat to eat.

> ANNA: You know, in childhood we always waited for my father to slaughter the reindeer. Do you know why? We were waiting with mugs to be filled. My father searched the carotid artery in order not to scare the reindeer. He petted and petted, and then a knife was stabbed into the animal exactly where he knew it to be done. But do you know what they are doing now?

Anna's face froze suddenly and became expressionless. Her eyes were wide open and she whispered as if she had memories and had witnessed brute violence.

> ANNA: They are using the hammer on the head of reindeer. Reindeer are scared, and the flesh is not the same. We eat, and something completely different is happening to health. Do you understand?

We nodded in response to Anna.

> ANNA: In the past! When we saw slaughtering in the past, when our parents were slaughtering, we never saw the raging mad eyes of the reindeer. Now during slaughtering I have seen the raging mad eyes of the reindeer. In the past the reindeer were treated as humans. People were talking with the reindeer. Now when I turn back to the slaughterhouse, I see the reindeer are treated as things. It's unbearable.
>
> I need to tell you why we were waiting with mugs. We drank blood, and then we made pancakes of blood. Nowadays there is no one who drinks blood. Such people are lost. They don't drink, because they feel unwell, they are not feeling well. No one wants to search the carotid now. And now there are unfamiliar, random people on the tundra. There is almost not any Sámi on the tundra. Our Sámi always showed respect and courtesy for reindeer. Yes, I tell very honestly. I am telling because I am suffering. I have pain in my heart.

I tell you now. Reindeer is what I really love. I have chosen the right way to go, and I have not lost the track. Do you understand?

We nodded.

The Pain of History

Anna opened her photograph album that lay in front of us on the table. She showed a photograph of a woman from the village of Voronja. The woman was leaning toward a cross, and her face was marked with pain. Anna said that the picture had been taken at a place of memorial for the homes, and all that was now covered with water.

> ANNA: My mother actually came from Kilginskii. It's a very old site. The authorities started to build railroads. Then those people came who wanted to have the reindeer, and they were stealing the reindeer. So then they moved to Voronja. Actually it is not a correct name, Voronja. In Sámi it's named Koarrdogk that means "full of streams." There were many streams. And now all of this is covered with water.
>
> And in 1961 and 1962 we had to move from Voronja, but they [parents] would not move. My parents stayed to the very end. They [the authorities] turned off the electricity, and food and mail stopped. We were forced to move from Voronja to Lovozero. The issue was that my parents stayed until the very last minute. They never signed their consent to move. Do you understand?"

Anna's face was expressionless. She was whispering, and her eyes asked if we could imagine what their not signing meant.

> ANNA: Violent!!! It was violent. All reindeer were taken to the state farm. We were forced to slaughter all the cows and sheep. We had private animals. In the Soviet period it was forbidden to have any privacy. We were therefore forced to move to Lovozero. The reindeers were taken from us and located on state farms. When we came to Lovozero, we were moving from place to place before we could settle.

We were moved from place to place, anywhere. For seven years we were dwelling in barracks.

"Were all displaced?" we asked.

> ANNA: Yes, forced. In two years...by us...Mother was living in silence for two years!!! And one day I was in the seventh grade I came home, and my mother was drunk. It was the eighth of March, the women's day. She was kneading dough. As usual she was baking perogies [dumplings] for the eighth of March feast.[8]

A festive day was transformed to a day of unhappiness.

> ANNA: Mother said, "I have a headache." She was bothered by headache. She said to my father, "I will have a nap. Please wake me up at 12 so I can continue baking." She never woke up. She was 47 years old when she died. She died on eighth of March, 1964, on the women's day. It's a date of broken heart. And my first husband died on eighth March, 2001. He was paralyzed for eight years. I was nursing him for eight years, and then he died.

Anna browsed the photograph album, and her first husband showed up on one of the pages. Anna said that her first husband started to drink heavily after their third child was born. It was difficult to live together with his heavy drinking. Anna gave him a chance time and time again and helped him up on his legs, but he was paralyzed from the alcohol damage and confined to his bed for eight years. Anna spoke about how she had nursed him and taken care of him without getting help from anyone—even though for many years she had opened her door and helped people who did not have a place to sleep because of the housing shortage and social suffering in the area.

Anna browsed the photograph album, and a faded picture of her father showed up.

> ANNA: My father had a hard fate. When he was nine years old, he was sold as a land worker.

Anna browsed further and pointed to a family tree that she had made after the damming of Voronja.

> ANNA: I have made a family tree, then I can remember. I have a very good memory. Voronchane, the people of Voronja are called Voronchane, they asked if I could create a map of the village. I have drawn all the farms.

"Was everything covered with water?" we asked. Anna nodded.

> ANNA: Everything was covered with water in the 1970s. We were forced to move in 1961, but the water came in 1970s. Then Voronja was covered with water. Can you imagine? I was...Mother died...Father said, "I can't live without her." He loved her very much. We went for a visit. Our houses were still there. Then I saw the houses were empty. At that time they were not covered with water. We were forced to move to Lovozero in 1962. In 1964 my mother died. In 1965 my father died. He could not live without her.

"How was your life after this critical event?" we asked.

> ANNA: Do you know? I was alone. We were three girls. I was the oldest one. I was 14 years old and had to work hard to keep the family together. I planted my own potatoes. I had to start the hard work of cultivating. It's the heaviest work. From the month of March on I was growing vegetables. It was beetroot, and when this was finished, there were carrots and cabbage to grow. I dried hay for fodder. During wintertime I worked with the animals and milked them. I milked the cows with a machine. Machine—milkmaid. But when the cows had calves, it was not possible to use a milking machine, and then I did it all by myself. Cows with newborn calves could only be milked with bare hands. Therefore my hands are broken.

Anna's hands were resting in her lap. Events in the past and present were woven together.

ANNA: The arms are worn out, they are tired. It feels like carrying heavy, heavy bags. I have been working all my life with helping others, helping sick people. My back is broken.

Anna raised her eyebrows and told us about the pain of loneliness and the exclusion from help when she was in a situation of need.

ANNA: And I remember that time I was starving. I was really hungry for several years. It was hard. There was no help, absolutely none. I remember it was not like that when we were living in Voronja. People were always helpful and very friendly to each other. There was always mutual help in everything. When Sámi had relatives in a poor condition, they were helping them. Now the Sámi people are not helping each other as they did before. Do you understand?

We nodded in response to Anna.

ANNA: And now I have sensed as soon as a Sámi family is in need, the new Sámi people keep a distance. There is nobody who cares. The Sámi people have changed. The new Sámi people are a completely different people. Do you understand?

Discussion

Anna remembered that in her home village, Voronja, Sámi people showed respect and courtesy to the reindeer. The reindeer were treated as *subjects*, persons to whom they talked and showed respect and dignity. This showing of respect for animals, and all living beings, was a matter of necessity in order to receive in return good gifts from the taiga and tundra. The Sámi way of acting toward others gave back good gifts and juicy reindeer meat.

Anna had experienced the new laws of the tundra: first the Soviet laws and then the laws of the money economy. The laws were experienced as violent acts toward the land and other living beings. Anna had witnessed the way that reindeer and the land were treated as things, *objects*, of the new and violent laws.

The new, violent way of acting toward other living beings resulted in dry local food without any juice, of reduced quality. A different taste, smell, and colour were experienced. The taste of the juicy reindeer meat and the fresh local foods that she remembered from her home village had been lost. Anna said, "We eat, and something completely different is happening to health."

The Cree in the Canadian Subarctic described what is happening to their health: "If the land is not healthy how can we be?" (Adelson, 2000). Adelson emphasizes that the experiences of a healthy land are connected to experiences of healthy bodies. Anna and the elderly Russian Sámi women in the ethnographic interviews experience loss of vitality and body moisture. Canadian Arctic indigenous peoples report loss of vitality, a decline in health and well-being, when they are unable to eat local food. These problems do not only emerge when climate change denies people access to local foods but are very much linked to problems associated with the undermining of local modes of production (Nuttall et al., 2005, p. 51).

I suggest that the experiences of dryness in local food (reindeer meat, berries on the ground) and bodies and of changed health are linked to what Veena Das has argued: the soul has left culture.

Culture and Soul

Anna asked several times if we could understand her, if we were following her story. It was not a question about our logical understanding, but rather asking if we were listening sensitively to the story, if we could imagine her emotional pain, her suffering in body and soul.

Veena Das (2007b, p. 40) says that pain is not inexpressible, not something that destroys communication or marks an exit from one's existence in language. Instead, it makes a claim asking for acknowledgement, which may be given or denied. The experience of pain cries out for the possibility of being heard, a response to the possibility that my pain could reside in your body, if only for a little while, and that the philosophical grammar[9] of pain is an answer to that call.

Inability to acknowledge the pain of others is apathy. *Apathetic* comes from the Greek word *apatheia*. *Pathos* means "emotion," and the prefix *a* means "without." For instance, emotionally distant fathers (parents) are not felt by their children to be present. They are emotionally absent, distant, or sceptical. Being emotionally absent toward others results not in a realization of my ignorance of the existence of the other but in my denial of that existence, my refusal to acknowledge it, my mental annihilation of the other. There is a violence that is not directed toward defending the self's integrity or rightfully demanding equality or freedom but expresses a wish for the other's non-existence. The failure to recognize pain is portrayed as a spiritual failure, not an intellectual failure (Das, 1995, p. 166).

Anna's eyes were asking again and again, "Do you accept my story? Do you want to hear? Do you follow me?" Anna asked us to listen sensitively to her story. In order to listen sensitively, we will discuss the Kola Sámi creation myth that was important to Anna.

Father Myandash: A Kola Sámi Creation Myth

In the Kola Sámi creation myth "Father Myandash, the Reindeer Man" we hear about the close relationship, the marriage between the reindeer man and the Sámi people. The Sámi and the reindeer are one body.

Common to all creation myths is their attempt to tell us who we are, what we are, or what we want to be. Creation myths are trying to interpret the mysterious and fabulous that we call our everyday life. In the book *Sámi Potato: Living with Reindeer and Perestroika* the two social scientists Robinson and Kassam (1998, p. 15) call attention to the reindeer as a metaphor for Sámi spirituality; they say that from it the Sámi derive meaning and cultural symbols. They make a structural analysis of the Myandash myth based on Levi Strauss's vertical and horizontal structures. Robinson and Kassam find the core of the myth and, as they say, an interesting message: even the best daughter and best wife might not be as good as reindeer or man. Myandash leaves his wife, taking along with him his now fully reindeer children, because of her misguided housekeeping practices. Clearly Reindeer Man knows best. So when conflict arises between Reindeer Man and the Sámi, the reindeer's desires should be closely heeded. The Myandash myth means simply that what is good for the reindeer is good for the Sámi. It is a statement of the very essence of Sámi life on the tundra lands of the Kola Peninsula (Robinson & Kassam, 1998, p. 22). Robinson and Kassam's analysis is based on ideas of binary oppositions where culture/nature, soul/body, and men/women stand in opposition.

Who Hears This Voice?

Awareness of violence, power, and gender are hard to grasp using models of binary oppositions. Violence and power dry out the soul of culture. Das argues instead that culture is born in the zone between, and it is in this zone that the truth about the culture can be spoken and heard (Das, 1995, p. 161). Culture as the adherence to socially proclaimed values dies when faced with the articulation of a voice from the zone between two deaths. From being a dead shell, culture births paradoxically at this juncture when a different relationship is established between hearing and the articulation of voice. This birthing is the act that enables us to speak of culture having a soul (ibid., p. 167). When a person can bear witness to suffering through the act of hearing, when the eye becomes transformed from the organ that sees to one that weeps, then we can speak of culture as having developed a soul (ibid., p. 162).

How Are We to Understand the Symbolic Language of Anna?

Anna spoke about events in the past in which she had learned to restrain undesirable emotions. She learned to express an image of being a good son. Jorun Solheim (1998) uses the term *the symbolic language of the body* in her book *Den åpne kroppen* (The open body). The experiencing world of the body is taken seriously. Solheim attempts to understand the experiencing world of the body as something that is communicated through a set of symbolic representations. The body speaks in images and analogies. Seen as a symbolic universe the body is not just nature but also a product of culture, a carrier of signs and meanings. However, because we are accustomed to considering the word, not the image, as a mediator of truth and reality, the symbolic language of the body might seem unreal and meaningless.

The experiencing world of the body is rich in metaphors and metonym. The hallmark of metaphors is the image, while the metonymic association

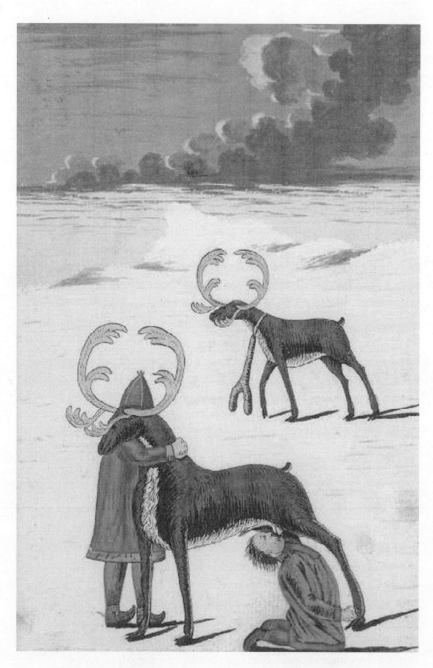

Sámi children drinking milk from a reindeer (Knud Leem, 1767). Photograph courtesy of Tromsø University Museum.

refers to proximity. One thing is represented by another that is commonly and often physically associated with it. Something is in contact with something else. We are facing two very basic ways of perceiving connections. Similarity and proximity are essentially based on sensuous bodily experiences and associations. The human mindset, our way of creating meaningful connection, is in some sense "magic" and is registered in these two basic forms of sensuous association (Solheim, 1998, p. 63).

In order to hear the voice of Anna, my Russian translator, Natalia, translated the very rich syambolic language used by Anna in her story (see note 5). Anna's father said *"Khorshaya synok"* to her, a female, because he emphasized that she, Anna, was his son: "Father said to me, '*Khoroshaya synok*,' you are a good son."

When Anna spoke about her experience of being a good son, her face became expressionless. She put intensity in her voice: "I said, 'From the fire.' I always said it was the smoke from the fire. I never told I was crying." Anna told what she did in order to fulfill her father's image of a good son. She restrained her tears and her desire for more than an inattentive father could give. Anna restrained her tears and her fears of being left alone. She worked hard and kept emotional pain in silence. The hard work of silencing emotions transformed her into being a good son.

Anna spoke about an ordinary moment in time when she had learned to endure and to do the hard work and all the everyday things that needed to be done. She learned to control emotions and weep in silence. Her father had left her alone with all the housekeeping, and he returned only after a long time, just as the Reindeer Man had in the Kola Sámi creation myth of Myandash.

Biographical Disruption

Anna had detailed memories of critical and traumatic events in her life. Her family was displaced from its home in Voronja in the 1960s. In the 1970s a dam caused their home and everything to be covered by water. Nevertheless, Anna had detailed memories.

The food memories from her home village were of clean, juicy, fresh, and diverse foods. There was a lot of food. The food was prepared in a way whereby it gave strength. The work of her mother transformed the food so that it tasted good. The recipe for her mother's fish soup and all the elements that were stirred into the soup in order for it to be good for human consumption were remembered in detail. Her mother said, "Everything in the soup is all what human's need." Gratitude, warmth, patience, solidarity, reciprocity, respect, and love are the essential and basic elements for the everyday life to be fulfilled. Many lovers of tasty food know that the person who stirs the pot has an impact on what is in the soup. The personality of the person who makes the soup can be tasted (Lupton, 1996, p. 32).

After the critical event in 1960, the displacement from their home in Voronja, Anna experienced a deep change in her everyday life. The way of acting toward others changed. Anna remembered from her home village the helping attitude that the Sámi people had shown toward each other and all other living beings. In her present everyday life Anna experiences a deep loneliness and social exclusion. She finds the new Sámi people very different from the Sámi people who had lived in the old Sámi villages. The new Sámi people are not helping others in need, as they used to do in their old settlements before the damming.

Anna experienced major changes and biographical disruption that caused illness and pain in her body. Pain was experienced in her heart, back, and hands. Vieda Skultans's (1999, p. 316) study of autobiographies from Soviet Latvia shows that major changes and biographical disruption influenced the women's perception of their own illness and sufferings. Illness narratives were interwoven with historical events and were seen as a logical outcome of the oppression by the state against every single individual.

Conclusion

Including a Kola Sámi woman's voice, so that it is heard, has brought an awareness of the health and illness experiences of marginalized people in the Russian Arctic. The voices of elderly indigenous women need to be listened to in Arctic health research. Paradoxically, health researchers are often in a position to inflict more suffering onto people by not listening attentively. It is important that health researchers accept the stories that people tell. The stories we hear can surprise, can be overwhelming or disturbing, and can be of such a nature that we otherwise would not like to listen to and consider them. As researchers we must ask an important question: Do we accept the stories that people tell? How do we write about the social suffering inflicted on women's lives as a consequence of social power? Das writes, "In repeatedly trying to write the meaning(s) of violence against women, I find that the language of pain through which social science could gaze at, touch or become textual bodies on which this pain is written often eludes me" (2007b, p. 38). In other words, there is no language in scientific texts for suffering.

In a time of major changes in the Arctic I find it essential to have a perspective that not only speaks to our intellectual understanding but also asks for our sensitive listening as social and health researchers. As social and health researchers we can learn sensitive listening from elderly indigenous people. The Sámi way of acting toward the other creatures of creation (even the berries on the ground) gives reason to claim that the command "Love your neighbour as yourself" (Matthew 22:39) should not be seen as only addressing human beings. Rather, our love should be directed toward the whole of creation (Jernsletten, 2010, p. 386). A Sámi theologian maintains: "In the age of climate crisis maybe we should see that it is through bending humbly towards the ground that we stretch toward the sky" (ibid., p. 387). I give the closing words to the Sámi philosopher Nils Oskal, as quoted by Jernsletten: "You must listen, be attentive. This is what it means to be a good human being—being responsible and taking care. This spirituality is not something ascending holy and apart from daily life, but a constant presence of other beings to whom you must be attentive. It is all about getting along with your surroundings. It is about an experience or stories about other people's experiences" (ibid., p. 388).

Author's Note

The author would like to thank the supervision and assistance of Rune Flikke, Associate Professor in the Department of Social Anthropology, University of Oslo; and Jon Øyvind Odland, Professor in International Health, Arctic Health Research, Department of Community Medicine,

University of Tromsø. Thanks go to Natalya Romanova for her translations and to all the Kola Sámi women who shared their stories.

Notes

1. The UNPF on Indigenous Issues (2012), *"Indigenous women and environmental violence": A rights-based approach addressing impacts of environmental contamination on indigenous woman, girls, and future generations* (paper submitted by UN agencies and indigenous peoples' organizations), http://www.un.org/esa/socdev/unpfii/documents/*EGM*12_carmen_waghiyi.pdf.
2. The leading international scientific body for the assessment of climate change. It reviews and assesses the most recent scientific, technical, and socio-economic information produced worldwide relevant to the understanding of climate change
3. The term dates back to Johannes Galtung and to the liberation theologians who used it to describe "sinful" social structures characterized by poverty and high degrees of social inequality, including race and gender inequality.
4. The Komi people live in the Republic of Komi, the Nenets Autonomous Okrug, the Arkangelsk Oblast, and the Murmansk Oblast. In the Russian Federation's legislation the Komi are not recognized as indigenous people, but in the Komi Republic's legislation they have that status. The Komi people face similar problems to those of other indigenous people in the Russian territories of the Barents Region: the loss of language and culture (www.barentsinfo.org).
5. Natalia, my Russian translator, translated *Khoroshaya synok* by finding words and technical help in a Russian-English dictionary. Natalia explains: "When the following words are said in Russian, *you are a good son,* both the adjective *(good)* and substantive *(son)* are masculine. In Russian it is *Khroshii synok,* but Anna's father says *Knoroshaya synok* because he emphasizes that *she,* Anna, is his son. He is therefore using the feminine for the adjective *(good)* and male for the substantive (son)."
6. *Loafkhess* (chive) was picked along the lakes and riverbanks or marshland. It was tied in bundles and put in fish soup (Bolsjakova, 2005).
7. The fish soup *Kull lumm* is a traditional Russian Sámi dish (Bolsjakova, 2005; Volkov et al., 1996). Bolsjakova (2005) describes the procedure: Half of the boiler is filled with fish, and water is poured in so that the fish is covered. Everything is boiled, and salt and onion are added to taste. The fish stock is poured into a mug and consumed. The fish soup is cooked when the eyes of the fish are white.
8. March 8 is celebrated in Russia with the making of perogies. For the feast the Russian Sámi make perogies filled with salmon, grayling, whitefish, reindeer meat (*puii vuennch,* a fat reindeer meat), and reindeer marrow. It should be "one

piece of fat." A Sámi fairy tale tells of a Sámi woman and her love for "a piece of fat." She does not need "the sweet" as tea, sugar, or sweet cloudberries, but she needs a piece of fat from the backbone of the reindeer (Bolsjakova, 2005).

9. The scenario to which Das is referring is Wittgenstein's question from *The Blue and Brown Books* about the way in which one's pain can reside in another body. "In order to see that it is conceivable that one person should have pain in another person's body, one must examine what sorts of facts we call criteria for a pain being in a certain place...Suppose I feel a pain which on the evidence of the pain alone, e.g., with closed eyes, I should call a pain in my left hand. Someone asks me to touch the painful spot with my right hand. I do so and looking around perceive that I am touching my neighbor's hand...This would be pain *felt* in another's body" (cited in Das, 2007b, pp. 39-40).

References

Adelson, N. (2000). *"Being alive well": Health and the politics of Cree well-being*. Toronto: University of Toronto Press.

Bolsjakova, N. (2005). *Žizn', obyčai i mify kol'skich saamov v prošlom i nastojaščem*. N. Romanova, Trans. Murmansk, Russia: Murmanskoe knižnoe izdatel'stvo.

Das, V. (1995). Voice as birth of culture. *Ethnos, 60*(3-4), 159-179.

Das, V. (2007a). The event and the everyday. In V. Das (Ed.), *Life and words: Violence and the descent into the ordinary* (pp. 1-17). Berkeley: University of California Press.

Das, V. (2007b). Language and body: Transaction in the construction of pain. In V. Das (Ed.), *Life and words: Violence and the descent into the ordinary* (pp. 38-58). Berkeley: University of California Press.

DiFruscia, K.T. (2010). Listening to voices: An interview with Veena Das. *Alterites, 7*(1), 136-145.

Farmer, P. (2004). An anthropology of structural violence. *Current Anthropology, 45*(3), 305-324.

Harris, A., & Guillemin, M. (2012). Developing sensory awareness in qualitative interviewing: A portal into the otherwise unexplored. *Qualitative Health Research, 22*(5), 689-699.

Ingold, T. (2000). *The perception of the environment: Essays on livelihood, dwelling and skill*. London: Routledge.

Intergovernmental Panel on Climate Change. *Climate change 2007 (AR4): Impacts, adaptation and vulnerability; Contribution of Working Group II to the Fourth Assessment Report of the Intergovernmental Panel on Climate Change, 2007*. http://www.ipcc.ch/publications_and_data/ar4/wg2/en/contents.html

Jernsletten, J. (2010). Resources for indigenous theology from a Sami perspective. *The Ecumenical Review, 62*(4), 379-389.

Kleinman, A., Das, V., & Lock, M. (1997). Introduction. In A.D. Kleinman, V. Das, & M. Lock (Eds.), *Social suffering* (pp. ix-xxv). Berkeley: University of California Press.

Kukarenko, N. (2011). Climate change effects on human health in a gender perspective: Some trends in Arctic research. *Global Health Action*, 4, 1-6.

Luk'jancenko, T.V. (1989). Lapps in the Soviet Union. In N. Broadbent (Ed.), *Readings in Saami history, culture, and language* (pp. 89-97). Umea: Centre for Arctic Cultural Research.

Lupton, D. (1996). *Food, the body and the self.* London: Sage Publications.

Mustonen, T., & Mustonen, K. (2011). *Eastern Sámi atlas.* Vaasa, Finland: Snowchange Cooperative.

Nuttall, M. (2005). Hunting, herding, fishing, and gathering: Indigenous peoples and renewable resource use in the Arctic. In *Arctic Climate Impact Assessment* (pp. S.649-690). Cambridge: Cambridge University Press.

Pink, S. (2009). Articulating emplaced knowledge: Understanding sensory experiences through interviews. In S. Pink, *Doing sensory ethnography* (pp. 81-96). Los Angeles: Sage.

Robinson, M.P., & Kassam K.-A.S. (1998). *Sami potatoes: Living with reindeer and perestroika.* Calgary: Bayeux Arts.

Sergejeva, J. (2000). The sun as father of the universe in the Kola and Skolt Sami tradition. In *Sami folkloristics* (pp. S. 233-253). Turku, Finland: Nordic Network of Folklore.

Skultans, V. (1999). Narratives of the body and history: Illness in judgment on the Soviet past. *Sociology of Health & Illness*, 21(3), 310-328.

Solheim, J. (1998). *Den åpne kroppen: Om kjønnssymbolikk i moderne kultur.* Oslo: Pax.

Volkov, N.N., Lasko, L.-N., Taksami, C., & Nordisk samisk institutt. (1996). *The Russian Sami: Historical-ethnographic essays*, vol. 2, Diedut. St. Petersburg: Russian Academy of Sciences at the Museum of Anthropology and Ethnography after Peter the Great (Kunstkamera), Nordic Sami Institute.

Young, T.K., Rawat, R., Dalimann, W., Chatwood, S., & Bjerregaard, P. (Eds.). (2012). *Circumpolar health atlas.* Toronto: University of Toronto Press.

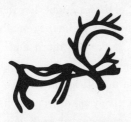

7

The Paradox of Home
Understanding Northern Troms
as a Therapeutic Landscape

MONA ANITA KIIL

It's just a natural thing, we don't talk about it that much. People know what they need to know. Traditional healing, being read on, it's just a natural thing.

Being a bit of Sámi, Norwegian, or a bit of Kven. It's a mix of people here; that's what we are, a mix, more than anything else. But it's nothing to talk about. (Thor, age 49)

Introduction

Thor reacted with slight frustration when asked about his relationship to traditional healing and the transcultural community in which he lives. He voices the dilemma that many experience in this context, namely, that of relating to practices that seem so natural but are experienced as utterly complex and challenging. As did most of the participants in this study, Thor also made a natural comparison between traditional healing and cultural identity, and these are therefore essential connections in this chapter.

The conventional outpatient clinic for mental health in northern Troms treats more than 400 patients a year. About half of these patients live in the municipality of Nordreisa, where the clinic is situated, while the remaining reside in the neighbouring municipalities of Skjervøy, Kåfjord, and Kvænangen. In addition to the conventional mental-health care, unofficial health care exists in many North Norwegian communities, consisting of traditional and religious healers whom people actively use or would consider using when faced with illness or crisis. Various traditional and religious healing practices are common in this area, and they go by several names depending on the locality. The main focus in this chapter will be on what is locally called *reading*, which is elsewhere known as *curing* or *blowing*.

In addition to cognitive psychotherapy, psychopharmacological treatment, and rehabilitation, the outpatient clinic offers art therapy and a generally open-minded attitude to the idea of integrating complementary and alternative treatment. Whether or not the clinic *should* have an actual integration of the local healing traditions is a much more complex question that will not be elaborated further in this chapter.

The main purpose of this chapter is to illustrate northern Troms as a therapeutic landscape and to portray its ramifications for understanding mental health in this region.

Initially I will give a brief review of the relevant literature in this field, followed by a presentation of the empirical background, method, and theoretical approach for this study, before employing passages from the story of one particular participant in the study, namely Johanna. Finally, by conceptualizations of Home, I will discuss themes made relevant in Johanna's story.

Background Review

In terms of research on health issues among the Sámi, the region of northern Troms is generally unexplored. In order to find relevant and recent research, one needs to look at the more typically Sámi research that often has its emphasis on the Sámi core areas of mid Finnmark. In general, research on health issues among the Sámi has primarily consisted of quantitative studies on somatic health, and the results for the Sámi are often compared with those of the majority population. The focus has been on health behaviour (e.g., Spein, 2008; Spein, Sexton, & Kvernmo, 2004), risk for disease (Nystad, Utsi, et al., 2008), and causes of death (Hassler, Johansson, Sjölander, Grönberg, & Damber, 2005). Research suggests that the Sámi do not face the same health-related challenges as do indigenous people in Canada, the United States, Russia, or Greenland (Symon & Wilson, 2009). Some researchers (e.g., Gaski, Melhus, Deraas, & Førde, 2011) have attributed the apparent absence of health differences between the Sámi and the Norwegian population to the acculturation processes. However, to my knowledge, the causal relations are more complex. In Norway, health services are largely public, which might contribute to higher levels of access to health services than in other countries (Hassler, Kvernmo, & Kozlov, 2008), and living conditions and educational levels are generally high. Nevertheless, research has identified several health-related challenges, such as Sámi-speaking patients being less satisfied than other patients with the services provided by municipal general practitioners (Nystad, Melhus, & Lund, 2008), and a study of mental-health care found that, compared with Norwegian patients, Sámi patients were less satisfied with their treatment and their contact with staff, and experienced poorer treatment alliance (Sørlie & Nergård, 2005). Self-reported health is poorer for the Sámi than for the Norwegian majority population (Hansen, Melhus, & Lund, 2010). Sámi individuals are more likely to experience discrimination and bullying than is the general population in Norway (Hansen, 2008), and discrimination is closely associated with elevated levels of psychological distress (Hansen & Sørlie, 2012). Not much research has been performed in regard to mental health and the use of traditional healing, with the exception of Olsen and Eide (1999), Kuperus (2001), and Sexton and Sørlie (2008), and the above findings suggest that merely looking at statistics is insufficient when grappling with (mental) health-care issues among people living in northern Troms. Even though being Sámi today is less stigmatizing than it was some decades ago, the process of developing an ethnic identity is still ongoing in many families, both in the Sámi areas and in areas like northern Troms. The loss of language and the confusion about ethnic identity may be associated with health outcome (Bals, Turi, Skre, & Kvernmo, 2010). Recent studies include the consideration of continuity and change within the Sámi world view in relation to the use of traditional healing practices (Kiil, 2013;

Miller, 2007; Myrvoll, 2010), people's relation to the traditional health-care systems in Sámi areas of southern Troms (Nymo, 2011), and the way in which Sámi people communicate in terms of health and illness (Bongo, 2012). Also, experience drawn from the Sensicam study (Kiil, Sexton, & Sørlie, 2010) indicates that patients within mental-health care in northern Troms prefer a qualitative dialogical approach when taking part in research projects, rather than responding to questionnaires.

Where the Three Tribes Meet: Ethnic Identity and Spirituality in "No Man's Land"

Troms and Finnmark are the most northern counties of Norway. Northern Troms covers a large geographical area, and the communities are sparsely populated. This region has been multicultural for centuries, populated by Norwegians, Sámi, and a small minority of Kven (descendants of Finnish-speaking immigrants to the area). In the coastal regions there is a greater proportion of Norwegians and people with mixed Sámi, Norwegian, and Kven heritage. Nordreisa is such a coastal community and thus the inter-section of three cultures or, as it is commonly referred to, "where the three tribes meet." Owing to the long-standing contact between the Sámi, Kven, and Norwegian communities many people have ancestors from all three ethnic groups. This is one of the reasons that the concepts of ethnic groups and cultural identity can be understood as complex and challenging in the region. The aim of the state policies before World War II was the assimilation of the Sámi and Finnish populations. Since the war the state policies have slowly changed from assimilation to integration. Of particular interest in this shift was the general interest in the concepts of roots and belonging, in the post-colonial Western world beginning in the 1960s and 1970s, and Sámi revitalization activism started in the same period (Eidheim, 1997; Gullestad, 1996). Another important reason for the complexity of the region is the varying degrees to which the assimilation policy has affected different geographical areas. The assimilation process was paralleled by individual experiences of stigmatization and discrimination (Eidheim, 1992; Minde, 2003; Thuen, 1995). For these reasons, people with Sámi ancestry in coastal regions may consider themselves as Norwegians today, and differences are not always obvious (Kramvig, 2005; Olsen, 2010). Many people might not identify with the symbolic expressions of a collective Sámi cultural heritage. Sáminess is thus often associated with the distant past and of little relevance to people's everyday lives (Gaski, 2008; Olsen, 2010).

In inland areas of northern Troms, Sámi revitalization was witnessed starting from the early 1960s (Mathiesen, 1990). In the coastal communities of Nordreisa and Skjervøy there has been no wave of revitalization as has been observed in the neighbouring municipalities of Kåfjord and part of Kvænangen. This lack of revitalization might be connected both to the distinct assimilation policies experienced by this area, as well as the nature of the collective identity that was promoted within the various municipal systems. The municipality of Nordreisa has a Kven Finnish profile; hence there is no official policy that supports Sámi identity or gives prestige to being Sámi. Festivals such as the Sámi indigenous Riddu Riddu in Kåfjord, the Verdde festival in Kvænangen, and the Kven Baski festival in Nordreisa can be seen both as expressions and manifestations of Sámi and Kven identity and as symbolic presences of the Sámi and Kven revitalization that has been taking place in this region. In addition to the cultural aspects already mentioned there is a particular spirituality attached to the region of northern Troms, on which I will elaborate in the following paragraph.

The religious awakening that today is known as Laestadianism was founded by the Swedish Lutheran minister and botanist Lars Levi Laestadius (1800-1861) and came to the northern parts of Norway from northern Sweden starting in the 1840s. Laestadianism spread through both Norwegian fishermen and the nomadic Sámis; in addition, the many Finns who immigrated to the north of Norway brought this religious movement with them (Kristiansen, 2005). Laestadianism was originally based on the teachings of Martin Luther but has through time been separated into different fractions, and some are known to be very conservative in regard to moral and theological issues. Although the Laestadians are members of the Church of Norway (Lutheran), the Laestadian congregations function as independent religious denominations. Laestadius, who also had a Sámi family background, was interested in the way in which the Sámi population managed illness and crisis in their everyday lives; he also referred to the healing traditions of the Sámi culture in his several books (Kristiansen, 2005). Laestadius, in contrast to Norwegian priests at the time, seemed to

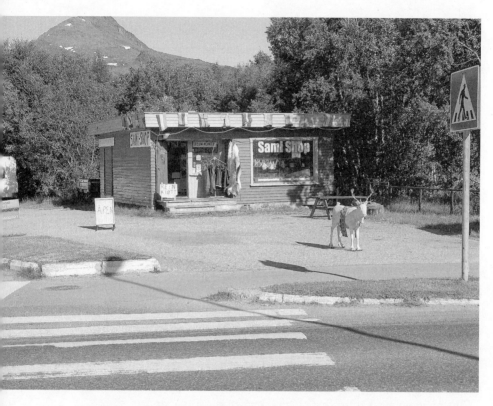

Within the region of northern Troms, Sámi culture is often portrayed as static and exotic, represented in this photograph of a souvenir shop in the municipality centre of Storslett.

have accepted the reading tradition, and in many ways this tradition corresponded with the solid foundation of the vivid and emotional spirituality that can be found in Laestadianism; although the latter might be understood as being more charismatic than the subtle reading practice, still they belong to a similar sphere of values.

Among the Laestadians of today it is fair to say that many are Sámi or Kven by origin, but there are also Laestadians who do not belong to either group or, as in the case of Nordreisa, are not necessarily aware of their ethnic heritage but all the same find a common community within Laestadianism. Laestadianism has in several ways erased the boundaries between the ethnic groups in this area; within the congregations the collective identity of Laestadian has been more strongly emphasized than that of the individual member's own cultural identity. The local healing practice of reading is an example of a phenomenon that is mutually influenced by the cultural and spiritual interactions in this region. Considering the fact that the conventional outpatient clinic for mental health in northern Troms serves the entire region, the factors mentioned in the next section can show how mental health and cultural identity are being managed at a general level, as well as the types of experiences and expectations that the patients individually bring into the consulting room.

The Practice of Reading: Communities of Care

Kleinman (1980) analyzes the way in which different communication systems interact, by using the concepts of popular sphere (here, the patients' local community), the professional sector (here, conventional treatment), and the folk sector (here, traditional practices). According to Kleinman's (1980) model of health and care systems, the traditional healing practices found in northern Troms belong to the folk sector, where one can find non-professional therapists who are closely connected to the local culture and world view.

Reading is commonly known as being a form of spiritual guidance and support during times of illness. It is a form of health care in the informal networks of these local communities, in which demonstrating awareness of each other's knowledge and problems plays a vital part. Reading performed by the reader is the speaking of Biblical words with the intention to heal. It is not the actual words that heal, but the power that comes with it. Reading is understood to be using God's power, not the healer's own energy. As one reader said, "I pray for the ill, and the rest is up to God, our father." The specific prayers used when performing reading are kept secret in order to avoid their being used by people not competent with the knowledge; also, importantly, the words are not revealed in order to maintain the ability to heal (Mathisen, 1989). There is a firm belief that a reader will lose his power if he is too public about his abilities or skills. The practice is hence of an implicit nature; it goes on quietly, and thereby not promoting the ability is an essential quality. When performing reading, the reader often uses tools that have natural elements, such as water, stones, soil, a knife, and paper.

Furthermore, reading is a kind of prayer directed toward a local and specific problem, and it is most commonly used for various emergencies related to illness and natural phenomena. The ability to stop blood or calm the sea has been closely related to the practice of reading (Henriksen, 2010). Reading can also be a path to soothe chronic illness, or it may have a more therapeutic function through the communication that arises between the reader and the one in need of help. It is not necessarily the one in need of help who contacts the reader; more often, family members, neighbours, or friends contact a reader on that one's behalf. This might be one of the reasons that the tradition of reading has been called a tradition of care or even a tradition of love (ibid.). Another reason is the fact that readers do not receive payment for their services; as one reader said, "what was freely given to me, I freely give." The term *reader* is more common than *healer*, which may be due to the fact that healing is often locally understood as a type of alternative medicine, while reading is defined as traditional medicine or folk medicine. Whereas the alternative medicine consists of a systematic training with the basic idea that anyone can be qualified to perform this method of healing, readers are considered to be naturally gifted. Readers may be autodidacts or have achieved their knowledge through training with a recognized reader or through older family members who have selected them to be the next carrier of these abilities. A reader has, at one point in life, somehow been given the experience or assurance that this is his or her duty or life task. Reading is considered to be a lifelong commitment, a calling. Regardless of this, the readers participating in this study seemed aware of their "shortcoming" in some areas and had no intention of competing with the conventional mental-health care. To my knowledge, they often advised their "patients" to see a professional doctor. "There is lots of suffering around," one reader said, "and our duty is to help the way we can, our way."

Material and Methods: Methodological and Ethical Considerations

This chapter is based on an ethnographic fieldwork conducted in Nordreisa from February 2011 to November 2012 among 12 patients who used the outpatient mental-health-care clinic for northern Troms. The material mainly consists of repeated in-depth interviews and participant observation. In total, 17 interviews were conducted, in addition to a number of conversations with readers, therapists, and staff at the clinic, people in the local communities, and locals living outside of the region. The participants were between the ages of 22 and 74 and included both genders. They were sampled on the basis of their interest in participating in the project and not by any specific diagnostic criteria. Regardless of this, all participants had been diagnosed with anxiety and/or depression disorders.

In order to follow up the core theme of the study, it was important to not make Sámi a narrow category but to approach the field broadly in order to grasp the diversity. Thus, a sampling based on patients acknowledging their Sámi or Kven background was considered problematic. None of the twelve participants clearly stated having Sámi or Kven ethnicity, and nine of them spoke about the feeling of being from a cultural melting pot, as Thor voiced in the introduction to this chapter. Seven of those nine participants did give the impression of desiring to acknowledge their Sámi identity. None of the participants stated a clear wish to acknowledge a Kven heritage; this could be explained through the somewhat interwoven position that Kven culture has achieved in Nordreisa, which has less controversy attached to it. As mentioned previously, the Sámi identity in Nordreisa is, to my knowledge, still more challenging and stigmatizing.

The interviews had an open-ended, yet semi-structured character, and an interview guide was used to direct the conversation to relevant topics regarding the patient's experiences. Semi-structured interviews help to produce specific answers to questions of concern (Spradley, 1980). This approach created a more informal setting for the conversation and encouraged the participant's own story to be highlighted. The aim was to develop a relationship of trust between the participants and the researcher and thereby obtain relevant data. The interpersonal interaction that arose during the interviews particularly, and the fieldwork generally, contributed to the production of knowledge as well as new problems for discussion. This can also be referred to as a symbolic interaction, and in the analysis of the data material it is therefore important to focus on the production of meaning as well as the production of content (Järvinen, 2005).

I discovered at an early stage that this project required a significantly different frame for doing fieldwork compared to the original idea of doing ethnography. First and foremost, it was ethically challenging to observe participants both in a clinical setting and in the privacy of their homes. My request of the participants in this study was that, when possible, our meeting should take place in their own homes or elsewhere outside of the clinic. Owing to a number of seemingly practical conditions, I met most of the participants at the clinic for the first time, and afterwards I met some of them in their homes. My original invitation to the participants, from the time we had met at the clinic, was for them to speak about the ways in which they as patients in this multi-ethnic context coped with their mental problems, and how they related to both the clinic and the traditional healers they had used.

Owing to the nature of these conversations, the use of a tape recorder sometimes felt uncomfortable for the participant. Even if recordings give accurate quotations, they might influence the conversation negatively; the tape recorder was used whenever the participant felt comfortable with it, and the data was transcribed verbatim afterwards. When a tape recorder was not used, handwritten notes were taken during the interview.

Data is not necessarily something one collects merely in the clinic or when interviewing participants. Rather, it evolves out of a process of learning and understanding—a socialization process. As such, it is also obtained through small talk and everyday events. Exploring and discussing various topics with the participants obtained much information and data. A large part of these informal conversations can be defined as ethnographic interviews, interviews in which one just lets information emerge without the need of prepared questions, pen, and paper. The flexibility of this approach makes it easier to have spontaneous interviews whenever the opportunity arises (Blaikie, 2000). In addition to ethnographical data, secondary data sources, such as historic files and relevant films, were used, as well as journals and newspapers covering the region.

As the participants lived in the four different municipalities that comprise northern Troms, one could say that this was a kind of ethnography by arrangement, in which interviews constituted the main method. The notion of *being there*—as an anthropological cornerstone—was therefore under some threat, and instead of being in the field permanently I found myself moving in and out of the field. Nevertheless, through my working on the project and staying in touch with the participants, the field was somehow incorporated in me and thus close and distant at the same time. Owing to the nature of this study, the ethnographic aspect could in some sense seem to be more an attitude brought into the project than an actual method. Regardless of this, the material left no doubt that the participant's story was the most important source of knowledge. I found these stories to constitute an ethnographic manifestation. Stories from childhood, stories from and by different generations where memories and conversations are central, also make the context; the field somehow moves beyond time and space. Marcus (2010) describes these as nested dialogues, a type of contextualized conversations. This kind of subjective reflection or para-ethnographic approach to life and society is increasingly becoming of vital importance in anthropological method, and it is a relevant starting point in order to grasp the methodological essence of this study.

It is crucial to bear in mind that encounters that move into the sphere of mental health are sensitive, and in terms of participating in a research project like this one, many of the patients can be said to be in a particularly vulnerable position. As a researcher one has to be prepared for the different emotional reactions that the interviews may evoke, and furthermore to reflect upon how one should meet such reactions. As a researcher I am a socially positioned person, who with my own cultural background and values participates in and influences directly or indirectly the way in which my participants respond, and potentially also may influence their lives. This was a challenge, contrary to typical clinical projects in which the researcher can relate solely to technical equipment or at least can have a more technical approach to the field. The project consisted exclusively of human beings, their stories, and the human interaction. On an ethical level this distinction is crucial and has often been mentioned in studies (de Vries, Anderson, & Martinson, 2006; Wagner, 1993) where so-called soft methods have been used in traditionally "hard" fields such as clinical medical practice. The study has received the approval of the regional ethical committee. The descriptions and quotations used in this chapter have been read and approved by "Thor" and "Johanna." All names have been given pseudonyms, and personal identification factors have been altered.

Home as a Theoretical Approach

Central in forming the analytical approach in this chapter is viewing *home* not as a fixed entity but, more dynamically, as a search for identity, which is an understanding of identity as something strategic, relational, and negotiable. According to Rapport and Overing (2007, p. 175), the concept of home has not figured much in traditional anthropological conceptualizations, except perhaps as a synonym for household (Carsten & Hugh-Jones, 1995). In that case, home was a stable physical space and a place that amounted to an "embryonic community" (Douglas, 1991, p. 289), in which territory and time were structured functionally, economically, aesthetically, and morally; so, even if the potential mobility of home was attested to—the tent of the nomad, say—the focus was still on the necessary routinization of time and space. Douglas elaborated that home could be defined as a pattern of regular doings, furnishings, and appurtenances and a physical space in which certain communitarian practices were realized. Homes began by bringing space under control and thus giving domestic life physical orientations—"directions of existence" (Douglas, 1991, p. 290). Furthermore, homes also gave structure to time and embodied a capacity for memory and anticipation. Thus, homes could be understood as the organization of space and time and the allocation of resources in space and over time. However, a broader understanding is possible and necessary and concerned less with the routinization of space and time than with their fluidity and with an individual's continuous movement through them (Minh-ha, 1994, p. 14). Rapport and Overing (2007) also explain that a conception of home is required that transcends the traditional ways by which identity is analytically classified and defined (according to locality, ethnicity, religiosity, or nationality), and is sensitive to allocation of identity that may be multiple, situational, individual, and paradoxical. As a concept, home must encompass cultural norms and individual fantasies, representations of and by individuals and groups; it must be sensitive to numerous modalities: memory and longing; the conventional and the creative; the ideational, the affective and the physical, the spatial and the temporal, the local and the global; both positive and negative evaluations (Wright, 1991, p. 214). As Simmel (1984, pp. 93–94) sums up, home may be said to provide a "unique synthesis" and "an aspect of life and at the same time a special way of forming, reflecting and interrelating the totality of life."

Johanna's Story

I have chosen passages of Johanna's story to represent this part of the material from the fieldwork in Nordreisa. Johanna's voice is in many ways the voice of all the participants because the topics she chose to make relevant in her story are also interwoven in the stories of the other participants. Johanna has suffered from depression and anxiety since she was around the age of 20. She has been in and out of treatment at the local conventional outpatient clinic for a number of years. Now, at the age of 57, she has returned to the clinic for treatment after several years of absence. When Johanna and I met at the clinic, she was focused on talking about her illness and her understanding of it. I have chosen not to pursue these aspects here. When telling her story in her home, Johanna shifts between talking about her own experiences with conventional mental-health care and those with traditional healers in this area, as well as referring to experiences of her relatives. She reminisces over her life as she paints a picture of Nordreisa.

It is late afternoon on a windy day in July when I arrive at Johanna's house. In her modest way of being, she welcomes me and shows me to her sitting room where she has arranged a small table with coffee and slices of lemon cake. She sends her husband outside to cut wood and store it for the upcoming autumn, and their dog follows him obediently. The house is quiet, yet the walls are all filled with photographs from Johanna's life: Johanna as a small girl in a yellow dress, giggling to the camera while holding a daisy; as a shy teenager hiding behind her classmates; as a blushing 1970s-style bride; and as a young mother holding her multi-dysfunctional daughter in her arms for the very first time. An old picture in a painted-photograph style of Jesus Christ receiving the Holy Spirit blends in with a number of photographs showing significant events from the lives of her now grown-up children that dominate the walls. In between there are pictures from magazines that have been framed, one of the late King Olav V of Norway, along with printed cards that contain words of wisdom; one card, overshadowing all the others, states, "Home Is Where the Heart Is."

Johanna's house is situated in a small area on the outskirts of Nordreisa where she has lived all her life. Her childhood home is just next door, but both her parents have passed away, and their house lies empty. The view from her living-room window includes the steep side of a mountain and a

rocky river running its course. The scenery is both breathtaking and potentially claustrophobic all at the same time.

My original invitation to Johanna when we had met at the clinic was to
speak about how she as a patient in this culturally diverse context coped
with her depression and anxiety issues, as well as how she related to both
the clinic and the traditional healers she used. On this day, however, her
story begins with memories of childhood.

> JOHANNA: I remember hearing Sámi words as a small child. It was
> like whispers in the wind... [Johanna smiles gently while she looks
> out of the window for a while.]
>
> I have this feeling it was my grandmother, on my mother's side,
> but I am not sure. We never really talked about these things in my
> family. It was sort of like a non-existing theme. My father did not
> want to hear about it; he used to say, "Just stop talking about this
> Sámi stuff." When I was a bit older I enjoyed being around the Sámi
> when they came down here in springtime, when they were moving
> their reindeer herds to summer grassland. It was always exciting,
> different; it sort of added flavour to our everyday life. They only came
> from the other side of the mountain, but I remember thinking that
> they were from another world. Growing up like this, with Karasjok[1]
> just over the mountain, I used to think that life was easier over there,
> clearer in a way. They sort of know more who they are...you are either
> Sámi or Norwegian here in Nordreisa, those things have always been
> so blurry, so hidden. These things became very clear to me when I
> was in my twenties; I was working in Finnmark and I really felt at
> home with the "Sáminess," it felt right to me, you know.

There is a warmth in Johanna's presence, and a poetic presence in her
words that gives an impression of confidence. Yet, even if she is the one
to raise the topic of cultural identity, and she speaks freely, she somehow
seems quite uncomfortable talking about it. When I confront her with this,
she admits that these are aspects of her life that she has not really talked
about before, and it makes her feel somewhat ashamed.

A Question of Knowledge

When we met at the clinic, Johanna did not go into detail about her experiences with traditional healers or readers; she only briefly mentioned them in answer to a question about whether she was familiar with traditional healing. She answered, "If you are in crisis or have problems, what I know works, no matter what, are the local healers and readers." I therefore asked Johanna at her home to tell me more about her relationship with readers. She answered:

> JOHANNA: Some of them I call, some I have visited in their homes. It's about people you know, that *know* something. If they are good, it always helps. You get names of good readers from others. Reading is something very familiar to me; it's like home. I have been used to it since I was a child, surrounded by it, one can say. I believe it's still common around here to see a doctor to get diagnosed and after see a reader to get cured.

Johanna talks quietly, with a sense of honour in her voice. She sometimes looks out the window or at her hands, where she plays with two silver rings. Other than that, she meets my eyes with hers.

> JOHANNA: There were no healers or readers in my family, though, but I think of myself as a kind of helper; but I am not a reader, no, I was not made out to be one. I just do what I can do—like pray for others; prayers work for me. I focus as hard as I can through thinking about the one in need; that's how I do it. It's not necessarily a Christian God I direct my prayer to; I don't really see myself as a Christian, even though I have kept my childhood faith. It's more like something spiritual; I don't feel the need to say it's like this or that. I have helped family members and a friend too, and they have been cured overnight, so to speak. Sometimes just minor health issues, other times more critical things. My sister is the one I have given most help to; she says I have warm hands. I also do laying on of hands sometimes, also with my daughter when she seems miserable or unstable. It calms her. One time my daughter was very unsteady; I

prayed very hard that night; the following day she was totally calm. I didn't actually think about it, not until seven months later. My daughter has abilities. She can see things before they happen. She just cannot communicate it through normal language. But I know that *she* knows that she has got these abilities.

Johanna shows that she is somehow self-empowered through her personal healing qualities, yet "dependent" on other therapists; she simultaneously helps and gets help from others, which, to me, bears witness to the encompassing quality of what I have previously referred to as a community of care.

Johanna clearly sees herself as being spiritual, but with regard to her religious belonging, there is a certain ambivalence:

JOHANNA: My grandfather was a Laestadian; he used to come over to our house on Sundays and preach to us. It was no fun...the radio used to be on, and you know, Sundays on the radio with violin music and church services and such...he always preached about us being sinners and about judgment day. Judgment day...oh dear God, still to this day I can't bear the sound of a violin. It was a heavy type of Christianity; as a child you got scared. My parents were not active in the congregation; they used to go for gatherings with my grandparents though, and then we had to go as well.

There Is a River Between Us

Johanna speaks about her long-lasting and, in her experience, challenging relationship with the conventional mental-health care:

JOHANNA: My relationship to the psychiatry has always been very tense. There have been far too many bad experiences throughout the years, disappointments. I have often felt let down; it has been like a struggle...You know, they are people educated to help...and then they end up making your crisis even bigger. It's difficult to explain really, but it's about understanding. You know when you feel ridiculed for doing things that are normal here, I mean things people do to manage, to comfort yourself or someone you care for. I mean, these things have been common here for centuries; people up north had to manage on their own. It's not like it's sorcery. Many doctors are, frankly, narrow minded, I tell you. They think it's only about superstition, and they don't see that this is helping many. It's like there is a river between us.

I ask Johanna to give me an example of something she would not share with the conventional therapist. She instantly refers to the time that she lost her father, a time that she was in treatment at the clinic.

JOHANNA: I was very close to my father, and when he passed away, I was in deep mourning for a very long time. When life is really bad, when I am truly struggling, I can sometimes feel the strong presence of my father. He comes to me in my sleep, but it does not feel like a dream; it's more like I actually see him. One time, I was awake, I saw him in a glimpse. My eyes were closed, but when I opened them again, he was still there. After a while he disappeared. This event gave me comfort in a time when my life felt like one big crisis. I spoke with a reader over the phone that very day. He made me feel at ease with that experience. I did not tell my [conventional] therapist at the time about this, though; I am not sure if I would ever be open about something like this. I mean, if you don't really trust them, you'll just end up using heavy drugs you don't really need. I know about totally sane people who have been diagnosed as lunatics because they have told about these things. For instance, if I should talk about my life and how I understand healing with most therapists the way I do with you, most will think I am totally crazy. But, I must say, this clinic is very good now; they seem to have an understanding of people here.

Johanna's being comforted by the presence of her late father can imply a world view or cosmology in which the everyday experience is only one of several potential realities or dimensions. These dimensions can be accessed through what is considered to be a sacred knowledge that exists within the various traditions. They may be accessed and become available for other reasons in the course of a person's life, sometimes in connection with crisis (Grieves, 2008; Vitebsky, 2003; Walsh, 2007). As Johanna said, this was natural to her and did not in any way reinforce her anxiety or depression; on the contrary, she felt very relaxed about it. One could say that the experience of her father's presence was consciously a part of Johanna's cultural narrative; when she is at home, she places it in a spiritual sphere, but when she enters the clinic, she removes it from her story for fear of presenting as psychotic.

Connecting with a Therapist

JOHANNA: For a long time I thought that I would never find a [conventional] therapist I would connect with. All that time I was acting as my own psychologist, I used different types of antidepressants; they were all really bad for me. It came to a point where I could not take it anymore; I desperately needed someone to help me. So that's when I came back to the clinic again, and everything is better now that I got to know Martin here at the clinic. He is different from all the other therapists I have ever met. I can actually be more of myself, if you know what I mean. Martin is from Nordreisa, he knows how things are here, but I don't think they have to be from here to be good therapists. What is important is if they have the understanding of what is normal here, so to speak. Just to be able to voice all these difficult thoughts, all this confusion, is a hundred times better than any medicine. The problem with most conventional therapists is that they are more focused on diagnosing you than listening to what you say.

The gap between Johanna's attitude toward and experiences with the conventional mental-health care, and her obvious need to simultaneously be part of it, seems at first glance to be a paradox. Judging from Johanna's story, one could draw the conclusion that the conventional mental-health care is not a necessity for her, considering the help she receives from readers. We could consider that, in order to be eligible for certain social welfare benefits, one depends on medical approval, but the participants never mentioned this factor as a sole reason for contacting the clinic. Five out of eight participants were also in full-time jobs, and according to them the need for a medical diagnosis for the social welfare system was not their reason for contacting the clinic. Even after connecting with the new therapist Martin, Johanna admits that she still holds back information from her therapist, in spite of the fact that this information could be helpful in her healing process or at least in managing her illness. Even as Martin is clearly trustworthy to her, Johanna still does not trust him enough to share certain parts of her story with him. Could it be that it is not merely a question of trust and alliance with the therapist but also the way that the patient chooses to draw her or his own boundaries in the clinical encounter?

Two Cultural Arenas: Home and the Unhomely

The arena of the clinic was somehow connected to the participant's illness narrative, while the arena of the participant's own home involved representations of the health narrative and matters concerning spirituality and identity. This could indicate that whereas the reader seems to answer a need for a local, spiritual anchor, the conventional therapist acknowledges the patient and his or her illness within the conventional system. However, the conventional system is the area to which people traditionally have not felt a belonging. There is also a collective orientation related to the practice of reading, while the conventional, clinical treatment is more focused on the patient as an individual. It may be equally important for the patient to be recognized in both regards.

Johanna draws a picture of a therapeutic landscape consisting of two different arenas in which people receive various medical treatments. It might be tempting to classify only the reading tradition as taking place in a cultural arena, but in my opinion the clinic must also be viewed as a culturally positioned arena. Conventional medicine can be seen as a strong representative of a Western world view, which therefore might seem particularly alienating for many patients in this context. In addition, one can say that psychiatry itself has its own embedded culture (Elgarøy, 2010) that can also be experienced as unfamiliar to Norwegian patients or culturally homogeneous patient groups (as compared to the more culturally diverse patients referred to in this study). Nevertheless, conventional mental-health care undoubtedly represents "the unhomely" for the participants in this study, which has been highlighted throughout Johanna's story. *The unhomely* is a turn of phrase coined by Bhabha (1994) that he employs to highlight the plight of the "unhomeliness" of all those people—refugees, migrants, the colonized, women, gays—who have no "home" within the (conventional) system. As of today, most indigenous peoples of the world also belong to this category. As a construct it refers to the state of hybridity— being neither here nor there—and as such it is situated within the post-colonial debate.

Despite my initial request to meet with participants in their homes many of them wanted to meet with me at the clinic, owing to practical issues such as travel distance or the need for public transportation. In the course of the fieldwork, however, it became clear that this was not merely a question of practicalities but also a manifestation of the way in which patients in this context have been "brought up" in the "conventional system." Through conversations with the director of the clinic, it became clear that assimilation policies contributed to the people in this area feeling accustomed to dealing with illness only in a clinical setting. This had implications, both methodologically and analytically, for how I was able to perform the fieldwork and how I could analyze and understand the material.

The question is, however, is this necessarily an experience of unhomeliness, or could it be understood as Johanna being at home in her untold stories? As Johanna having no need for sharing her innermost, spiritual encounters? As her story making authenticity and homeliness for her and those close to her? Can withdrawal of information in fact be a construction of home for people like Johanna? Is the information that she chooses to keep apart from the therapy a key factor of who she is—the difference that makes the difference, her identity? Johanna does not need to share these sides of her story, because they are and should continue to be implicit. This can be a recognition that the homes of many remain invisible, and that home comes to be located in different ways, as it does in memories and myths and in stories carried around in one's head. Practices and narrations that do not merely tell of home represent it and serve as cognitive homes in themselves. According to Rapport and Overing (2007), and as Bachelard (1994) puts it, the human imagination always builds "walls" of impalpable shadows, comforting itself with the illusion of protection, and so carries "the notion of home" into any "really inhabited space," whether cognitive or physical. A paradox of home can also be that it is by way of transience and displacement that one achieves an ultimate sense of belonging. According to Kateb (1991, p. 135), to be at home "in one's own place" it is necessary to become alienated and estranged to some degree, mentally or spiritually. For Hobsbawm (1991, p. 63), exile is a resource inasmuch as it gives that vantage point from which one is best able to come to know oneself. It is for this reason too that home "moves" us most powerfully as absence or negation.

Through Johanna's story one can see that home can also recall ambiguity and that even the homely can be experienced as alienating, for example in the strict rules of Laestadianism to which she was exposed as a child. A working definition for charting the morass of ambiguities and fluidities of contemporary identity as shown through Johanna's story may therefore be of home as "where one best knows oneself" (Rapport & Dawson, 1998), where "best" means "most," even if not always "happiest." Perhaps not only can one be at home in the ambiguity of culture, but that ambiguity itself can be one's very home; as Thor stated in the introduction, "we are a mix, that's what we are."

Conclusion

The field research that formed this chapter focused on how an ambiguous historical context has created a certain framework for understanding identity, and how users of an outpatient clinic in northern Troms experienced being between two significantly different medical and cultural systems. Johanna's story is therefore shown to be not only a narrative of self or illness but also a narrative that can contribute to the understanding of home, an analytical concept.

The idea of home can, for patients like Johanna, represent the ability to juggle between these two medical and cultural worlds, that is, to juggle without being misinterpreted or misunderstood in the clinical setting for their use of traditional healing practices such as reading. As users of traditional healing practices such as reading, the participants in this study who are represented through Johanna experienced a significant sense of vulnerability in their encounter with the conventional mental-health service.

They expressed lack of trust in the conventional mental-health service with regard to the way in which their traditional and religious practices were being understood. Among other factors, they feared being misdiagnosed with more severe mental-health disorders if they should communicate their personal treatment philosophies. In communities like Nordreisa, where there are complex and coexisting health paradigms, various barriers to trust can be caused by both the patient's own boundaries in the clinical encounter and the professional interpretation of his or her traditional healing pathways. In such contexts an awareness of the patient's transcultural position should be included in clinical practice to make conventional mental-health care more patient centred.

Author's Note

I would like to express my greatest gratitude to the participants in this study, who have so bravely shared their stories and their time with me. I thank the outpatient clinic for showing open-mindedness to the study. My heartfelt thanks go to the traditional healers with whom I have been in touch, and to other participants in and from the local communities of northern Troms. Thanks go to the Norwegian Research Council for financially supporting my doctoral project, "Cultural Perspectives on Mental Health in Northern Troms"; to the Psychiatry Research Group at the Department for Clinical Medicine, UiT The Arctic University of Norway; and to its leader and my supervisor, Professor Tore Sørlie, for support.

Note

1. Karasjok is a town with a significant Sámi population in the county of Finnmark. Even though the municipality of Kvænangen is situated between Nordreisa and Karasjok, Nordreisa is in a straight line with Karasjok, and participants often referred to Karasjok as a place "over the mountain."

References

Bachelard, G. (1994). *The poetics of space*. Boston: Beacon.

Bals, M., Turi, A.L., Skre, I., & Kvernmo, S. (2010). Internalization symptoms, perceived discrimination, and ethnic identity in indigenous Sámi and non-Sámi youth in Arctic Norway. *Ethnicity and Health, 15*(2), 1–15.

Bhabha, H.K. (1994). *The location of culture*. London: Routledge.

Blaikie, N. (2000). *Designing social research*. Cambridge: Polity Press.

Bongo, B.A. (2012). Samer snakker ikke om helse og sykdom: Samisk forståelseshorisont og kommunikasjon om helse og sykdom; en kvalitativ undersøkelse i sámisk kultur [Sámi people do not talk about health and illness: Sámi understandings and communication of health and illness; a qualitative study of Sámi culture]. Doctoral dissertation, University of Tromsø, Norway.

Carsten, J., & Hugh-Jones, S. (Eds.). (1995). *About the house*. Cambridge: Cambridge University Press.

de Vries, R., Anderson, M.S., & Martinson, B.C. (2006). Normal misbehaviour: Scientists talk about the ethics of research. *Journal of Empirical Research in Human Research Ethics, 1*, 43–50.

Douglas, M. (1991). The idea of a home: A kind of space. *Social Research, 58*(1), 287–307.

Eidheim, H. (1992). *Stages in the development of Sámi selfhood*. Oslo: University of Oslo.

Eidheim, H. (1997). Ethno-political development among the Sámi after World War 2. In H. Gaski (Ed.), *Sámi culture in a new era: The Norwegian Sámi experience* (pp. 29–61). Karasjok, Norway: Davvi Girji.

Elgarøy, S. (2010). Om kulturen i psykisk helsevern [About culture in mental-health care]. In A. Silviken & V. Stordahl (Eds.), *Samisk psykisk helsevern: Nye landskap, kjente steder og skjulte utfordringer* (pp. 16–33). Karasjok, Norway: CalliidLagadus.

Gaski, L. (2008). Sámi identity as a discursive formation: Essentialism and ambivalence. In M. Minde (Ed.), *Indigenous peoples: Self-determination, knowledge, indigeneity* (pp. 219–236). Delft, Netherlands: Eburon.

Gaski, M., Melhus, M., Deraas, T., & Førde, O.H. (2011). Use of health care in the main area of Sámi habitation in Norway: Catching up with national expenditure rates. *Rural and Remote Health, 11*, 1655 (online).

Grieves, V. (2008). Aboriginal spirituality: A baseline for indigenous knowledges development in Australia. *Canadian Journal of Native Studies, 28*(2), 363–398.

Gullestad, M. (1996). *Everyday life philosophers: Modernity, morality and autobiography in Norway*. Oslo: Scandinavian University Press.

Hansen, K.L., Melhus, M., Høgmo, A., & Lund, E. (2008). Ethnic discrimination and bullying in the Sámi and non-Sámi populations in Norway: The Sáminor study. *International Journal of Circumpolar Health, 67*(1), 97–113.

Hansen, K.L., Melhus, M., & Lund, E. (2010). Ethnicity, self-reported health, discrimination, and socio-economic status: A study of.Sámi and non-Sámi Norwegian populations. *International Journal of Circumpolar Health, 69*(2), 111-128.

Hansen, K.L., & Sørlie, T. (2012). Ethnic discrimination and psychological distress: A study of Sámi and non-Sámi populations in Norway. *Transcultural Psychiatry, 49*(1), 26-50.

Hassler, S., Johansson, R., Sjölander, P., Grönberg, H., & Damber, L. (2005). Causes of death in the Sámi population of Sweden, 1961-2000. *International Journal of Epidemiology, 34*(3), 623-629.

Hassler, S., Kvernmo, S., & Kozlov, A. (2008). Sámi. In T.K. Young & P. Bjerregaard (Eds.), *Health transitions in Arctic populations* (pp. 148-170). Toronto: University of Toronto Press.

Henriksen, A.M. (2010). *Å stoppe blod: Fortellinger om læsing, helbredelse, hjelpere og varsler* [To stop blood: Stories of reading, healing, helpers, and signs]. Oslo: Cappelen Damm.

Hobsbawm, E. (1991). Introduction. *Social Research, 58*(1), 65-68.

Järvinen, M. (2005). Interview i en interaktionistisk begrebsramme [Interview in an intractionist conceptual frame]. In M. Järvinen & N. Mik-Meyer (Eds.), *Kvalitative metoder i et interaktionistisk perspektiv* (pp. 27-48). Copenhagen: Hans Reitzels Forlag.

Kateb, G. (1991). Exile, alienation, and estrangement. *Social Research, 58*(1), 135-138.

Kiil, M.A., & Salamonsen, A. (2013). Embodied health practices: The use of traditional healing and conventional medicine in a North Norwegian community. *Academic Journal of Interdisciplinary Studies, 2*(3), 483-488.

Kiil, M.A., Sexton, R., & Sørlie, T. (2010). Sensicam (cultural, self-help, and CAM sensitive psychiatric treatment approach: An interventional study). Unpublished research protocol.

Kleinman, A. (1980). *Patients and healers in the context of culture: An exploration of the borderland between anthropology, medicine, and psychiatry.* Berkeley: University of California Press.

Kramvig, B. (2005). The silent language of ethnicity. *European Journal of Cultural Studies, 8*(1), 45-64.

Kristiansen, R. (2005). *Sámisk religion og læstadianisme* [Sámi religion and Laestadianism]. Bergen, Norway: Fagbokforlaget Vigemostad & Bjørke.

Kuperus, K. (2001). *Kartlegging av behovet for tilrettelagte helse: Og sosialtjenester for det samiske folk på Helgeland* [Mapping the need for adapted health and social care for the Sámi people in Helgeland]. Hattfjelldal, Norway: Sijti Jarnge.

Marcus, G.E. (2010). Notes from within a laboratory for the reinvention of anthropological method. In M. Melhuus, J.P. Mitchell, & H. Wulff (Eds.), *Ethnographic practice in the present* (pp. 69-79). Oxford: Berghahn.

Mathiesen, P. (1990). Ethnicity as pattern: Past and present. *Acta Borealia, 7*(1), 5-13.

Mathisen, S.R. (1989). Faith healing and concepts of illness: An example from Northern Norway. *Temenos, 25*, 41–47.

Miller, B.H. (2007). *Connecting and correcting: Case study of Sámi healers in Porsanger.* Leiden, Netherlands: CNWS Publications.

Minde, H. (2003). Assimilation of the Sámi: Implementation and consequences. *Acta Borealia, 20*(2), 121–146.

Minh-ha, T. T. (1994). Other than myself / my other self. In G. Robertson, J. Bird, B. Curtis, M. Mash, T. Putnam, & L. Tackner (Eds.), *Travellers' tales: Narratives of home and displacement* (pp. 8–26). London: Routledge.

Myrvoll, M. (2010). *"Bare gudsordet duger": Om kontinuitet og brudd i sámisk virkelighetsforståelse* ["It is only the word of God that counts": Of continuity and rupture in Sámi understandings of reality]. Doctoral dissertation, University of Tromsø, Norway.

Nymo, R. (2011). *Helseomsorgssystemer i samiske markebygder i Nordre Nordland og Sør-Troms: Praksiser i hverdagslivet* [Health care systems in Sámi communities in northern Nordland and southern Troms: Everyday practices]. Doctoral dissertation, University of Tromsø, Norway.

Nystad, T., Melhus, M., & Lund, R. (2008). Sámi speakers are less satisfied with general practitioners' services. *International Journal of Circumpolar Health, 67*(1), 114–121.

Nystad, T., Utsi, E., Selmer, R., Brox, J., Melhus, M., & Lund, E. (2008). Distribution of apoB / apoA-I ratio and blood lipids in Sámi, Kven, and Norwegian populations: The Sáminor study. *International Journal of Circumpolar Health, 67*(1), 69–83.

Olsen, K.O.K. (2010). *Identities, ethnicities, and borderzones: Examples from Finnmark, Northern Norway.* Stamsund, Norway: Orkana Akademisk.

Olsen, T., & Eide, A.K. (1999). *Med en klype salt: Håndtering av helse og identitet i en flerkulturell sammenheng* [With a pinch of salt: Managing health and identity in a multi-cultural setting]. Report 9/99. Bodø, Norway: Nordlandsforskning.

Rapport, N., & Dawson, A. (Eds.). (1998). *Migrants of identity: Perceptions of home in a world of movement.* Oxford: Berg.

Rapport, N., & Overing, J. (2007). *Social and cultural anthropology: The key concepts.* London: Routledge.

Sexton, R., & Sørlie, T. (2008). Use of traditional healing among Sámi psychiatric patients in the north of Norway. *International Journal of Circumpolar Health, 67*(1), 135–146.

Simmel, G. (1984). *On women, sexuality, and love.* G. Oakes, Trans. New Haven, CT: Yale University Press.

Sørlie, T., & Nergård, J.-I. (2005). Treatment satisfaction and recovery in Saami and Norwegian patients following psychiatric hospital treatment: A comparative study. *Transcultural Psychiatry, 42*(2), 295–316.

Spein, A.R. (2008). Substance use among young Indigenous Sámi: A summary of findings from the North Norwegian Youth Study. *International Journal of Circumpolar Health, 67*(1), 122–134.

Spein, A.R., Sexton, H., & Kvernmo, S. (2004). Predictors of smoking behaviour among Indigenous Sámi adolescents and non-Indigenous peers in north Norway. *Scandinavian Journal of Public Health, 32*(2), 118–129.

Spradley, J. (1980). *Participant observation.* New York: Holt, Rhinehart, & Winston.

Symon, C., & Wilson, S.J. (2009). AMAP *assessment 2009: Human health in the Arctic.* Oslo: Arctic Monitoring and Assessment Programme.

Thuen, T. (1995). *Quest for equity: Norway and the Saami challenge.* St. John's, NL: ISER Books.

Vitebsky, P. (2003). From cosmology to environmentalism: Shamanism as local knowledge in a global setting. In G. Harvey (Ed.), *Shamanism: A reader* (pp. 182–203). London: Routledge.

Wagner, I. (1993). A web of fuzzy problems: Confronting the ethical issues. *Communications of the* ACM, *36*, 94–101.

Walsh, R. (2007). *The world of shamanism: New views of an ancient tradition.* Woodbury, MN: Llewellyn Worldwide; London: Routledge.

Wright, G. (1991). Prescribing the model home. *Social Research, 58*, 1.

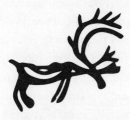

8

Keeping Doors Open
Everyday Life Between Knowledge Systems in the Markebygd Areas

RANDI NYMO

Introduction

One of the regions in Norway populated by Sámi is called the Markebygd (woodland rural districts) region. Some of the districts are situated in the northern part of Nordland County, and others in the southern part of Troms County. In this region many of the Markebygds form communities that cut through municipalities and counties. In the rural societies where the Sámi have lived, and still live, the governmental policy of Norwegianization has run parallel to the program of modernization. However, in spite of hard Norwegianization efforts, the dwellers of these districts have kept their Sáminess. The Norwegian language has not replaced the Sámi language everywhere, and core elements of the culture are still intact (Nymo, 2011). As an insider, born and raised in one of the Markebygds, I can attest that the Sámi culture has not disappeared. There has been a "new-figuration" of culture, as Rossvær (1998)[1] calls cultural development, when there has been a meeting of "old times" and "new times."

The Markebygd dwellers are many faceted in their ways of meeting everyday challenges, as evident in areas ranging from industrial activities to health and illness practices and circumstances. A fair analysis of the practices in the Markebygds does not permit a forced conformity with standard Western relevance and causality thinking. I realized this during the data production for my doctoral thesis (Nymo, 2011). It struck me that the informants in the study often interpreted and explained their experiences of daily life as fated or having arisen from imbalances that could cause health problems and illness. In their minds, the imbalance could be a disturbance caused by bad spirits or by bad wishes from other persons. It was understood that good relationships between persons were important to avoid illness. The informants also seemed to be "experts" in navigation, creating space for managing situations. This is a practice within a model of thinking called *birget* (finding ways to do, to manage, in Sámi) (Nymo, 2011). It is a model of Sámi life philosophy described by Kalstad (1997) that reflects Sámi thinking as practised in reindeer husbandry. The *birget* model searches repertoire for handling each situation.

Background

The assimilation policy of the Norwegian state was conceived and implemented from the mid-1880s and executed by different means toward the midst of the twentieth century. Some attempts had already been implemented during the previous millennium, such as christening the Sámi.[2] Shamanism was forbidden, and the Sámi were deprived of the instruments for practising Sámi religions. An example of that systematic work was the organized collection by the authorities, the Church included, of shamans' drums, from Salten in Nordland County to Namdalen in Trøndelag County, and their transportation to rectories where they were received by the clergymen. For the occasion they had engaged skilled old Sámi to explain the figures on the drums (Dunfjeld, 2006). Without tools, the possibility of practising religion was reduced and eventually negated. Additionally, *joiking* (chanting song, in Sámi), being associated with shamanism, was forbidden. This contributed to a gradual shift in religion. The Norwegianization imposed by law from the 1880s onwards further managed the work. The children were forbidden to speak Sámi at school. The primary school law of 1889 directed all schooling to be done in the Norwegian language (Christensen, 1997, p. 99).[3] Additionally, the use of language was controlled during the children's recesses (Andersen, 1999; Nymo, 2011). In the same way, owners of land were forced to take Norwegian surnames. In the Markebygd areas, where many of the Sámi had staked out a future as small farmers after losing their reindeer, and because the local trend was to be settled, almost all Sámi names were eliminated as a result.

The new life brought change to the local dwellers on many counts. The implementation of Norwegianization, and its overall supervisory control, categorized Sámi cultural traditions as primitive and inferior. This resulted in the stigmatization of Sámi as second-class humans, reinforcing the view that a "new thinking" should replace "the old fashioned" one. The Markebygd people were offered, as were other Sámi, new practices for their everyday living, and from the late-nineteenth century they were put under some pressure to accept them. When there was resistance among the Sámi, and simply being Sámi was seen as resistance, it was often characterized as an attempt to stop modern development (Drivenes, Hauan, & Wold, 1994; Minde, 1997). Therefore, the awareness of differences gradually appeared in social interactions. Realities could split family members and relatives, and some districts were regarded as more modern than others. However, it is a long distance from Oslo to the Markebygd region, and each area was exposed and affected in various ways. The phenomena of backstage and front-stage (concepts of Goffman, 1992) seemed to be available for practising the Sámi language. In some homes, families, and local communities the Sámi language continued to be used, at least in the arenas where it was possible. Other locals followed completely the directives of the Norwegian authorities, and corrected the people who still spoke Sámi. Norwegian public officials (such as teachers, health personnel, agriculture bureaucrats, and priests) administered the laws, but they did so personally and according to the situation (Nymo, 2011).

The Use of Indigenous Philosophy

The Norwegianization and modernization processes gradually led to changes in basic patterns of thinking, as the prohibition on practising Sámi religion had an influence on cosmologies. Ontologically we can talk about objective and subjective positions. Epistemological grounds are influenced by these ontological positions. An example of the Sámi ontological approach is the understanding of nature as having its own force and spirituality. Being born into a culture informs one's epistemological ground and leads to the ways and means of learning; that is, knowledge leads practice. In short, epistemology determines the way to handle challenges in everyday life.

A useful theoretical instrument for my work of understanding and contextualizing Sámi traditional healing has been a model illuminated by Foley (2005) on indigenous philosophy. In this context, philosophy means world view, cosmology, or systems of beliefs, in which indigenous philosophy looks upon the world as a trinity of the physical world, the human world, and the sacred world. The physical world includes the earth and everything living; the human world consists of human beings, knowledge, relationships, and practices; and the sacred world is responsible for the mind (spirit) and cultural traditions (Foley, 2005). Understanding practices in the frame of indigenous philosophy is also interpreted by Berkes, Colding, and Folke (2000) and by Helander-Renvall (2008). Indigenous philosophy and indigenous knowledge are considered by Smith (1999), Verran (2005), Nakata (2007), and Porsanger (2004, 2010) to be linked to each other. Practising knowledge is based on thinking or philosophy and ties an individual to her or his society (Rolf, 1995). Personal knowledge also functions as a broker between the personal interests of an individual and her or his fellowship. Rituals and rites are often common instruments for practising personal knowledge, and help to navigate the challenges of everyday life. The use of rituals, for instance, helps the individual to remember how to behave in nature, and by remembering rites one can be aware of changes in the ecosystems (Berkes et al., 2000). Curing by the use of folk medicine is the practising of traditions, and being able to practise requires the remembering of rituals. In that way the individuals are tied to incorporated knowledge, brought forward from generation to generation. Rituals and rites, in the way they are used by indigenous people, are incorporated knowledge.

To sum up, traditional and cultural knowledge have a basis in cosmology, ontology, and epistemology and influence the understanding and interpretations of phenomena in everyday life. This leads to the finding of suitable practices to meet challenges. When the Sámi culture, religions, and language were suppressed, the ways to think, practise, and speak were challenged. In addition, when the majority culture was comprehended as the modern and more developed one, and the Sámi experienced that their ways of thinking and doing things were seen as primitive and even unlawful, it is understandable that it was considered best not to speak openly about this thinking or philosophy and to hide the practice of this indigenous knowledge. Doubtless, it was painful to have ancestral practices trampled underfoot by the claims of modernity.

Playing Roles in Managing Daily Life Activities

There are residual processes today from the time of extensive Norwegianization. These processes show the consequences of the pressure placed on the Sámi culture, language, and world view or philosophies and are the underlying tensions within local Markebygd societies. The tensions result from the early modernist movements in which a stigma was put on the Sámi during the time of assimilation, but they can nowadays be expressed unconsciously by the Sámi themselves in different situations; one such case is the elimination of the open use of personal knowledge. The tensions have also led to mixed blessings; for my generation in particular, multi-resource practices have led to a level of prosperity. The mixed blessings are very visible for the generation of my parents: on the one hand, they pushed their children to get an education and, on the other hand, they complained that they should not forget their Sámi heritage. My parents' generation did an exceptionally valuable balancing act. They continued to uphold the traditional thinking and knowledge that was brought forward by their parents but adapted with new thinking. This balancing has been worth gold for my generation in strengthening the position of Sámi culture.

This chapter discusses the ways in which Markebygd Sámi balance the living of daily life when confronted with the demands made by the Norwegian "cultural recommendations." This balance and work can be associated with individual role-playing, as construed by Goffman (1992). Playing roles, according to Goffman, can supply the interactions with flexibility and stability. Inside the playing of roles there is predictability and memorized mechanisms to prevent the undermining of stability.

Extended Kinship Influences Health-Care Systems

The Markebygds have a strong social network, constructed by kinship and neighbourliness (Nymo, 2011). Kleinman (1980) has explored sectors of health-care systems and suggested a model based on studies of the intersection of health-care systems in Taiwan. This has helped me to understand Sámi kinship as a power in daily life. The structure of Kleinman's model of a local health-care system includes three sectors: the popular sector, the folk sector, and the professional sector. The popular sector is the largest one, and Kleinman suggests that this sector is important but poorly understood. Patients leave the professional sector to be taken care of by members of the popular sector. The folk sector is classified into sacred and secular parts. For the Markebygds, making a sharp distinction between the popular sector and the folk sector does not always clarify the local practice; their consulted practitioners are often within their families. Families, relationships, and regional societies seem to foster their own healers (Nymo, 2011). Kleinman's study shows that folk medicine in Taiwan is related to both the popular and the professional sectors. In the Markebygd societies a connection is not made between folk medicine and the professional medicine's arenas in Norway. Operative in the Markebygds are strong kinship relations, forming an expressive popular sector, which have occurred as an institutionalized arrangement (Nymo, 2011) strengthening the popular sector, and treatment given in the sector is often supplemented with healing from folk medicine's practitioners.

Methodology, Fieldwork, and Interviews

The empirical data for this text is taken from my doctoral work and was collected in 2006–2007 (Nymo, 2011). Additionally I use data collected for my master's degree (Nymo, 2003). Therefore, the data used in this text will be analyzed for a second time. Such an additional analysis widens the use of a researcher's own data in such a way that new data is produced, and some phenomena can be brought to a new understanding. Moreover, existing theories will be supported, and new knowledge generated (Thorne, 1993; Wicklund, 2008).

The data produced has come from written material, stories told about daily life in the Markebygds, and from my own observations. I did fieldwork at organized gatherings for elders and people with health failures, on a monthly and theme basis, as arranged by the Sámi Cultural Centre, Várdobáiki, in the municipality of Evenes in north Nordland County. The participants came from the Markebygds in the municipalities of Evenes (north Nordland) and Skånland (south Troms). I focused on how the participants (including the leader and the speakers) interacted with each other and on what was said about chosen themes. Observations included, for example, the ease or difficulty with which participants brought forth their thoughts and feelings. I was interested to observe how the discussion flowed, and certainly I was a participant observer. My fieldwork also included patients from Markebygds in their interaction with medical personnel during their stay in the local hospitals in the towns of Narvik and Harstad. At the hospital I was directly observing and not participating.

From these different locations (Várdobáiki and the local hospitals) informants were recruited for interviews. The informants from Várdobáiki were strategically chosen from the participants, and I met them in their homes. Interviews at the hospitals were conducted in connection with and after the observations. The interviews focused on the challenges of living at the intersection of Sámi and Norwegian cultures during and after the time of Norwegianization. I was presented with stories about lives in prosperity and in adversity. A number of stories focused on the daily life that was marked by the situation in which the one culture (Sámi) was less valued than the other (Norwegian) by the authorities. The stories told were many sided, and in spite of suppression they expressed cultural richness and good ways to *birget* (manage) living in the Markebygd culture.

Data Production and Analysis

The analysis is based on hermeneutic phenomenology (van Manen, 2007) and Goffman's theories of micro interactionism (Goffman, 1974, 1983, 1992). The analysis does not rigidly make themes or categories. Life stories, according to van Manen (2007), are about lived experiences and are difficult to bring to a form of conceptual abstraction. However, phenomenological themes can be interpreted as structures of experiences (van Manen, 2007).

Prior understanding worked side by side with the theories to interpret the data. Common cultural codes expanded the researcher's search for meaning in the stories told by the informants, leading to a comprehensible context and an organizing completeness. An example of how cultural codes helped to structure phenomena from the field that was lived experience can be illustrated by the following. Returning home from the field in my car, I reflected on the gathering of informants as a cheery group. They were frivolous. Being frivolous (*lettliva*, in Sámi) in this case showed qualitative well-being. I am familiar with this understanding; to be frivolous carries value in the Markebygds. With this realization one phenomenological theme can be explored: stories, humour, silence.

In that way a hermeneutic phenomenological theme structured my work. As Nakata (2007) has said, indigenous researchers ought to be upgraded as knowledge holders. I have been a "knower" during many situations of my research. Sometimes I have added my own experiences to the text with the intention of widening the horizon of understanding. With reflection on the theme of "stories, humour, silence," the concept of situational moments appeared in the analysis. At the health gatherings I observed that storytelling was welcomed. The contents of the stories were, as usual, about phenomena experienced by someone in the Markebygds. After a story had been told, the participants recollected its events, and they could have different understandings of the story. I observed that some of the participants had a humorous approach, while others responded silently to the same story, told by one or another.

Such portraits were welcomed differently by the participants. However, there seemed to be ample space, in the way of speaking and listening, for the participants to achieve a compromise. Humour was often used as a vehicle to bring the situation to a common agreement, even as the participants seemed to avoid actual conflict in the discussion.

Ethical Considerations

The study was performed inside a territorial enclave, and therefore the data has been strongly depersonalized. The stories are mixed, such that one informant's story is spread among several fictive persons. My data deals with human life experiences and thoughts, and the material has a personal and partly sensitive character. The intention is to complicate the identification of persons.

Another ethical consideration is that qualitative studies often attempt to arrive at the meaning behind the spoken words of the informant (Foss & Eilifsen, 2004). The researcher wants to come as near to the informant as possible and therefore often crosses the border of his or her private sphere. The project has also navigated to picture the way in which the informants have managed their Sáminess in small districts. Some of the stories told by informants are about others. These are the ethical dilemmas of using narratives to which Osgood (2010) calls attention. Before its commencement the project was approved by the regional ethical committee for medical research ethics in Northern Norway. As a secondary analysis often seeks new meanings and new points in the material, I also contacted the committee before initiating the secondary use of the material, and it raised no objections.

A Situation

Inga is an old woman living in one of the Markebygds. I met her during the work on my master's thesis. She welcomed the Sámi cultural renaissance in the 1970s and 1980s, and her clear Sámi language represented both potential and active help for many young people who were trying to regain their lost language. Many young people visited her home to ask for advice and means. She also managed to sew Sámi costumes (*samekofte*) in accordance with the local tradition. She had taken care of her mother's *samekofte* and used them as models for new costumes. However, Inga, being a confessioned Laestadian Christian, faced a dilemma. In the beginning of the Sámi cultural renaissance there had been considerable local resistance from the Laestadian community against Sámi politics and the cultural bloom. The Laestadian preachers considered faith and Sámi ethno politics to be antagonists. It almost seemed as though they thought that engagement in Sámi cultural work could displace the Christian faith.

When I interviewed Inga, she said that she would have liked to wear her mother's costume in the 1970s as well as now. She said, "I want to dress in my mother's *kofte*, but I dare not and I don't want to do that." So on the one hand she longed to dress herself in her mother's *samekofte*, but on the other hand she did not know if she really wanted to wear the costume. Here she demonstrated a double standard or the holding of two opposite norms.

I will now discuss three possible models for understanding Inga's behaviour. First, I will put it in the context of Bateson's (1973) double-bind model, in which Inga's ambivalence can be considered as a form of split communication. As a psychiatric nurse I am familiar with Bateson's double-bind theory as a form of "schismogenetic" communication. Such a form of communication contributes to ambiguity and confusion and can be comprehended as pathogenic. During the course of my psychiatric work and in interaction with Sámi patients I have abandoned Bateson's theory. I arrived at an adjusted view through my experience that Sámi patients were clearly not comfortable presenting their case histories to the health personnel; they tried to behave as "good Norwegians," which often resulted in actively hiding their Sáminess. The non-Sámi health personnel, knowing that the patient had Sámi heritage, interpreted in terms of a double bind these communications that evaded clarity on being Sámi, which I now see as a mistake. However, in spite of having grown up in a Markebygd, I also could often go too easily with the flow of my colleagues.

The second model is a local popular understanding. According to Mathisen (1989), local non-Sámi considered the Markebygd Sámi as unreliable people. Norwegians living near the Markebygds had learned that the Sámi tried to hide their Sámi ethnic identity in interactions outside the Markebygds. The local non-Sámi made an obvious misinterpretation, that of unreliability, in not understanding that the Markebygd Sámi may have had good reasons for hiding their Sáminess that in no way indicated unreliability.

Certainly the one-sided use of theories can lead astray. I found that neither the scientific double-bind model nor the popular unreliability model
had enough explanatory power. My preliminary conclusion when using
the two models was that the Markebygd Sámi were locked in inflexible
models of interpretation. But then a third possibility proved to be more productive. During my doctoral work I figured out, with the help of Goffman
(1983, 1992), a third possibility to interpret and analyze Inga's presentation
concerning her mother's Sámi costume. As a methodological situationist
Goffman acknowledges that every interaction has its own logic. That indicates that the interaction contains an internal logical steering, whereby the
actors mutually agree to let the situation be brought to an end (Aakvaag,
2008). Goffman (1983) explains that interactions and role-playing are working together. Success in this work affirms that the actors have to define
common frames. In this construction the society can be seen as a collection
of situations.

In a context of methodological situationism Inga's ambivalence can be
interpreted as two different situations. As a Laestadian woman she preferred to follow the recommendations of the community. She therefore
never dressed in her mother's *samekofte* or other Sámi costumes. Inga was
faithfully practising her religion. The other situation was that she started
to sew Sámi costumes for the young Sámi activists. They were able to wear
traditional local models of the costumes in meetings with Sámi from other
areas. Inga's engagement was a contribution to maintaining the cultural
tradition and providing Markebygd youth with correct Sámi costumes. Inga
solved the emergent dilemma by putting into practice both an acceptable
religious behaviour and her Sámi cultural activity.

By using Goffman's theories of methodological situation and the way
that people present their selves in everyday life, one can interpret Inga's
ambiguous behaviour in the context of the management of situations and
challenges that are the consequence of hard Norwegianization. One consequence is seen in religious practice. Even though Laestadianism is called
the Sámi religion, there are adaptations and interpretations of the texts
whereby connections to the older Sámi religious thinking are avoided.
Basically Sàmi cultural expressions were avoided because the older Sámi
traditional religion had been labelled unchristian. In the Markebygds
the Sámi women found that wearing colourful clothing to Laestadian

gatherings could be taken as an eye-catcher and a disturbance to the Christian message's reaching the members of the congregation. The Sámi women gradually avoided wearing clothes coloured in the traditional red, yellow, green, and blue (Minde, 1997). Another consequence of the hard Norwegianization was a lack of practical sewers of Sámi clothes. This lack occurred during the Sámi culture's rise. Inga did something to balance this lack until the young people themselves were able to produce *samekofte* and Sámi-inspired clothes.

A Way to Manage Face-to-Face Interactions

Goffman (1974) uses the concept of frames to make clear that people in interactions have to define every situation in an attempt to understand each other. It is important to have a common understanding of what is occurring. A common understanding requires a common frame. To succeed in making a common frame for interaction, the participants have to "read" the situation and adjust to it. That means that people in face-to-face interactions have to choose how they should behave in order to, according to Goffman (1974), provide clues for keeping up the interaction. After having defined the situation, they attempt to do the right things, to behave in a way that is suitable for the defined frame.

In the Markebygds, where Sámi lived close to Norwegians, they had daily interactions. The Norwegianization and modernization called for, as I have mentioned before, the Sámi to behave as good Norwegians and suppress that they were Sámi. In spite of these precautions, however, the Norwegians, as a rule, mentioned in meetings with Sámi that the Sámi were not real Norwegians but actually primitive Lapps[4] from the woodland who were visiting the community centres. All authorities, offices, and shops were located usually about one Norwegian mile (10 kilometres) from the Markebygds. To manage the necessary interactions, the Sámi had to speak the Norwegian language, and the level of ability to express their errands in the Norwegian language differed among the Sámi actors. Often they themselves knew that they spoke with a characteristic Lappish accent. They learned that they were considered to be primitive, and they developed tactics to succeed.

A man told a story at a meeting,[5] in which I was a participant, about how the Markebygd children learned to do the shopping for their mothers in town even though they knew they could be attacked by Norwegian youths. In wintertime they skied to do these errands, but they dared not bring skis to the shop because the skis could be disturbed while the children were inside the shop. They hid the skis under trees at the graveyard. When they arrived at their destination, the shop owner, a woman, locked the door behind them. The man remembered that she was a kind woman who helped them to state their needs, to pay, and to pack their sacks, and then let them out. They would take off at a high speed, often with the Norwegian youths close behind. The Markebygd youths were good runners, and as a rule the Norwegians were left behind. When they reached their skis, they knew they were safe because they were even better skiers than runners. Gradually they could pass without attacks, but they never fully trusted the Norwegian youths.

The man told this story proudly. When analyzing with Goffman's frame theory, one can deduce that the story is an example of how the Sámi used their skills as skiers to achieve acknowledgement. Negotiating successfully with the Norwegian youths gave freedom of action as well as access to the community centre, which also was the centre for the Markebygds in that particular part of the municipality of Skånland. Perhaps they used the graveyard as a hiding place because they reasoned that it was esteemed as a holy place for all actors and therefore it ought to be a free zone. The man's story does not say anything about how they managed to do this kind of errand for their mothers during the summertime. As an insider I know that during the summer the husbands were free to go to the town and they used bicycles. During the wintertime the husbands were often away for work, fishing in Lofoten. The fishing brought food for themselves and their families, as well as earning them money from the companies for which they fished. The men could also be away from home for roadworks, for example, which was relief work arranged by the authorities. From my own experiences I know that we were ordered to do such duties when our fathers were away for seasonable work during the winter. My mother, for instance, used to write a message to the teacher to let me be free every Friday to visit the food store for the weekend shopping, when I was a student at junior high school. We were mixed together with Norwegian students. The man's age is about half a generation more than mine, and his generation was not offered school outside of the Markebygds.

Managing Norwegianization

Another story I want to present, illustrating that the framing of situations was necessary to keep the daily life going during the time of Norwegianization, was told by two elders from a Markebygd about their school time. They are about 80 years old now. When they were pupils at elementary school, the law forbad the use of Sámi language in school and its close surroundings. Teachers, often from the south, had to see that the rules were followed. However, the Markebygd children were not perplexed. Longing to use their mother tongue during free time, they waded over a river at recess. There the teacher could not hear them speaking Sámi, and they neglected the teacher's call for the next lessons. They also knew that the teacher was not able to cross the river because he had no suitable footwear for such an exercise. They wore Sámi footwear (*komager*), prepared with a mixture of tar and oil, and the *komags* were tied with bands around their legs to avoid water getting inside the footwear. The informants emphasized that they were good jumpers from stone to stone and that they knew the easiest crossing of the river. This went on for some weeks, but then the situation was turned; the teacher was provided with a flute. They could neither ignore the sound of the flute nor continue to prolong the recess. The informants comprehended that a line for acceptable behaviour had been drawn and that they had to accept the rules.

We see how the children played with frames so that situations were easy to handle. They fetched help from the landscape, and their bodies knew how to behave in the landscape. The landscape helped the Markebygd children, and thus being able to negotiate was a part of the education. The teacher seemed to understand the children's situation and was co-operating. It was preferable to create a good atmosphere to achieve new goals in raising Norwegian-minded children. It is not unreasonable to think that the teachers who proved successful in the work of Norwegianization were rewarded. In Finnmark during the 1890s teachers were promised an increase in salary if they succeeded in implementing a conscientious Norwegian state education program for Sámi and Finnish pupils (NOU, 1995, p. 6). Such reward could also be rendered as honour.

In about 1930 the Norwegian state program for schools stated that good food traditions were required for better health among Norwegian children and youths (Oslo kommune, 1932). An attempt was made to implement this idea over the whole country, including schools in Sámi areas. The two informants from Markebygds remembered that their teacher bought fish oil and porridge oats and involved the children in the plan for good health. The two informants remember that they did not like the taste of fish oil. To get rid of it and instead of drinking the liquid, they used the oil to grease the *komags*. The *komags* became more and more waterproof. The informants reflected during the interviews, wondering if the teacher had realized what they were doing, spoiling the expensive fish oil. We can think that the teacher chose to neglect their behaviour because the smell of fish oil ought to have told him that they did not swallow it. Perhaps he did so because the situation in which he had involved them depended on the pupils' willingness to co-operate.

The school did not have sufficient funding to buy fish oil and porridge oats. So to accomplish the health program, new negotiations between the teacher and his pupils had to take place. They had to develop frames for new situations. The informants said that the teacher asked them to pick berries for sale and that if they brought berries to the school, he would find buyers. The children saw a chance to be out during the school day. In the forest and on the hills they were allowed to speak Sámi. They had footwear to be outside, and their traditional knowledge was a capital in which to frame the school time. The informants remembered one highlight very well: their school was elected as the best school in the municipality. This gave the pupils and the teacher a big boost and was welcome.

Today, particularly during the summertime, when the Markebygd adults who have moved away from their "childhood land" are staying for vacation, they often meet and recollect their childhood memories and share their experiences of school days. They assumed that they had had to put up with the realities of Norwegianization and do their best in every situation. They could not sit down and mope and trouble their parents, who, they knew, had enough worries about managing their existence in Markebygd areas. Their parents had to tackle meetings with Norwegian authorities within domains such as agriculture, house building, church systems, and health services. The informants knew that their parents had to manage a "rugged" and unknown terrain. Their parents had to understand the atmosphere of the interactions in which they were involved, and so work on their arguments.

Goffman as a methodological situationist acknowledges every inter-action's own logic, a logic that does not detract from the attributes of the participants or social structures (Aakvaag, 2008). According to Goffman (1983), the participants in interactions are playing roles, and therefore it is necessary to provide the situation with a common frame, and this includes the clarification of roles. In this context the society is thought to be a series of social situations (Aakvaag, 2008). When analyzing the material, I wondered if that assumption was valid for all the situations in which the informants in the study were involved. For those who were the actors, clarifying roles seemed to be important for the outcome of the interactions. Perhaps, some were better role players than others and quickly imagined the situation and turned it to the best, making a common frame.

Traditional Knowledge Challenges Modern Ways
Believing in Complementary Treatment

One situation in which the informants particularly encountered world view and practices colliding with modern ways of thinking and practising was the meetings with the health and agriculture services. There they met some actors who were friendly disposed, while others are remembered for their unfriendly behaviour. First, I will discuss the interactions with actors of the professional health service, and, next, the meetings with the local agricul-ture services.

Most of the informants who told of meetings with members of the health services remembered both curious and rude comments from physicians about their use of traditional treatment. An old man spoke about his neigh-bour who had hurt himself with a saw while preparing wood. The neighbour called a traditional healer, *læsar* (reader, in Norwegian), with the intention of stopping the bleeding, just as he always did before going to a physician. The *læsar* also had knowledge to limit the pain. When the cut was under control, and the man felt well, he went to see the physician. The physician asked, "Have you lost much blood?" The man answered, "No, I have seen my neighbour who has knowledge to stop bleeding." The physician continued, asking, "Do you have or have you had pain in the sore?" The man answered, "No, my neighbour removed the pain." The physician then said with a gruff voice, "Do you really still believe in that old-fashioned thinking?" The man knew that the time had come to not say any more about the issue and to let the physician do his work. The man also thanked the doctor for his analgesic and promised to come back if the sore became infected. He paid, went home, and followed up with his neighbour's "expert help."

The informant indicated that, by asking the man if he still believed in such old-fashioned treatment methods, the physician had generalized Markebygd people as a congruent group, in accordance with old stigmas. My informant reflected with me over the phenomenon that Norwegians in many cases often lump everyone together when they refer to one person's practice in the Markebygds. It appears as a way to delineate the ethnical border between the population on the coast, where Norwegians live, and the people in the uplands, where the Sámi live. We can also ask whether the physician and health personnel are amazed that traditional medicine is still in use among the Sámi. Mathisen (2000) calls attention to certain competitive conditions between folk medicine and professional medicine near the end of the nineteenth century. The old medical reports tell of a campaign to prevail over folk medicine, expressing the opinion that the people had a lack of knowledge and that they continued to get help from miracle men and quack doctors (Løken, 1900; Mathisen, 2000). According to Mathisen (2000), modern medicine promoted the idea of having a moral responsibility to intervene and lead the people to a good understanding of health, illness, and treatment. Going deeper into the material, it can be understood that the medical actors intended to control the field. By the way in which the physician commented on the man's account we wonder whether the professional medicine is speaking defensively, admitting failure to dominate. The health-science actor recognizes that the patient tells him about the use of a folk medicine practitioner without any dishonour. It has been a practice among the Markebygd people to try to hide their use of healers when visiting medical doctors, but they have not been successful. This has caused questions from the doctors, sometimes experienced by the Sámi as being degrading to their Sámi integrity. This Markebygd man does not hide the use, and in that way he avoids further discussion. The medical doctor does not need to pump information from his Sámi patient; he gets clear information immediately. Could it be because the Sámi man has been socialized to make the best of interactions between the Sámi people and the actors from the Norwegian health-care system when situations come to a head? Perhaps it is an implicit frame, in which experienced phenomena are bodily engraved, and this engraving helps him to navigate in new situations that remind him of earlier experiences. I would say that Goffman's theories (1974, 1983) about bringing situations into balance work for this situation. Furthermore, the Markebygd man is not forbidden to use folk medicine. One interpretation can be that it is acceptable to combine treatment methods. In addition, the man has his network in the Markebygd where he can tell about his encounter with the physician. Typical for people having a strong popular sector is the nearness to helping instances. There is always somebody to listen and share experiences. The popular sector of health-care systems explored by Kleinman (1980) takes care of daily life challenges, and works to encourage individuals.

When Farming and Care for Farm Animals Impinge on Modern Thinking

On the small farms there is a long tradition of helping each other. It seems that it has been better to join forces than to struggle alone. Being together enabled ongoing communication and shared information. For example, an initiative was made to cultivate grain during World War II. Together they created food supplies for their own safety. An informant spoke about how his parents and their neighbours started grain production during the war and sowed oats and barley. It was hard work from start to finish, and they had to trust in help from each other. Together they bought a thrashing machine. The machine was shared, transported from one small farm to another, and followed by an operating crew. To keep the machine in operation, manpower was needed. This could be accomplished because it became a joint project, and creative thinking, a kind of knowing, was involved—the kind of creative thinking that is called *birget*, in which there is management of common initiatives, and resources are applied to facilitate subsistence farming.

After the war, implementation of the programs of Norwegianization and modernization started, including the modernization of small farms, such as those in the Markebygds. The land of the Markebygds was cleared for new ground, and cultivation began, with the intention of providing better crops of grass. The ideology was that the small farmer should concentrate on agricultural work and not be a multisystem worker. Combined industries should be ended in favour of specialized agriculture. Therefore, the collective systems were challenged; every farmer had to manage for himself. Many felt locked into a strange system. They had, for instance, to report when a piece of a field was cultivated, and then they received a subsidy. When the authorities import rules for the Sámi, this is in itself a break in the cultural way of behaviour (Helander, 2004). What happened in the Markebygds has parallels in other Sámi areas; the subsidies were not easy to resist.

Another change in everyday life was that the common grazing lands for the animals ceased to exist, and only cultivated pasture connected to the farms was in use. Again the collective thinking was put under pressure. It had been the children's tasks to bring cows and heifers to the common pasture, and now a good transmission of knowledge between adults and children, and also among these groups, was broken. This was serious, because the transmission of practical personal knowledge between individuals is dependent on these close interactions. To view the consequences we can call on Rolf (1995). He showed that traditional knowledge and its practices tie communities together. The new time brought splits to the collective thinking in the Markebygds and promoted more individualistic persons. New conflicts emerged between neighbours when the animals grazing in a field broke the fence and crossed over into a neighbour's cultivated land.

We can still ask, however, whether the new claims eradicated indigenous philosophy or thinking. A story told by an informant concerns illness among farm animals. The informant is a man of about 80 years of age. His memories were from his best years as a farmer. He had a cow that could not stand up after calving. They tried to tie a rope around the body of the cow and hang her up on a hook, but the cow was so weak that she fell down. The owner called the veterinarian, who came. After some inspection he declared that the man had to put the cow to death. The farmer was disappointed. The veterinarian had advised what was considered to be a radical act. The farmer knew about a traditional folk healer, *læsar*, living in the parish next to his, and that same night he walked through the darkness to discuss the situation with him. The *læsar* considered that the cow could be saved. He read some rituals onto a piece of black wool thread and instructed the farmer to tie the thread around the cow's left back foot and let the thread stay there until it fell off. The cow recovered and continued to live without any further problems, and produced much milk. The winter passed, and one day while the farmer was out in the fields doing spring work, the veterinarian, having an errand in Markebygd, stopped his car and came to the fields to talk to the farmer. He wanted to express his regrets that nothing could have been done to cure the cow when he had been called. Then the farmer answered, "The cow is living very well, and she is fine and fit." The informant said that the veterinarian had a look of disbelief but said nothing. The farmer invited him to come and see the cow, but he did not want to. Afterwards this farmer had difficulty in getting the veterinarian to turn up if he needed expert help. The veterinarian would answer his query with an angry voice, saying, "You can fetch your own veterinarian, the Svartfors–dyrlegen [Blackwaterfall veterinarian]." This answer is similar to the answer given by the physician in the previous story, with a certain dismissal and resentment. The message so given seemed to be that the Markebygds ought to follow the non-Sámi advice and only employ knowledge from Western medicine.

To sum up, we can say that after the war it was necessary to follow the advice of the agriculture authorities to increase production and prosperity. And it was a way to have an easier everyday life. The Sámi could concentrate their employment, and the economy became stabler. The women also had an easier daily life because the small-farm work was not handed over to them and the children when the men had to work outside the farms. They used the extra time to do humanitarian work and brought additional health management to the small societies; for instance, there were new child health programs in which local women worked together with public health nurses and physicians (Nymo, 2011). In that way the Markebygd people participated in creating the promotion of health. However, as we have seen, the Western medicine philosophy did not eliminate the folk medicine and did not get the upper hand.

Nature as a Subject

One of my informants was a woman staying in one of the two hospitals that were in my field of study. During our conversation she told a story about her husband, from his childhood in a Markebygd. They were both about 50 years old at the time of the interview. They both had stable jobs and participated in leisure activities. When he was a child, he used to have bad thoughts, and he would not talk about these to his parents. He felt that his mother had so many worries in her daily life, and he wanted to protect her. His father was there, silent and hard working. The boy used to go to the forest, and there he ventilated bad thoughts. He met and talked to *ulda* (little people, in Sámi). He experienced the characters, who revealed themselves as kind and helpful. In this experience we see that the landscape and nature are more than simply a place for recreation. The young man found an encounter that was helpful to him against his mental restlessness. He expressed or unloaded bad thoughts onto the *ulda*, which became a sort of container. In the Sámi culture, *ulda* are characters who may reside at any location, and when they are met, people ought to interact with them. They often appear in dreams, or one can have a feeling that they are around. They always have a message. I will illustrate *ulda*'s activities with a story told by an informant (Nymo, 2003). The informant told about fetching wood in a forest. He used to follow his grandfather for that work, during which they would stay overnight in a bunk cabin. One night the informant heard indeterminable sounds, like people talking. He was afraid, and the grandfather said, "Don't be afraid. It is only *ulda*, and if we do not disturb them, then they let us in peace." In that way the young man learned that one is never alone wherever one goes. The clue is to learn to sidestep the phenomena, not to cause injury to them or to oneself.

A story from my family tells about negotiating with *ulda*. The story is well known, having been told from generation to generation as well as outside of my family and kinship.[6] It is about my great-grandfather, John Hansen, and his work in a little forge that he had as an additional industry on his small farm. He used to work in the forge at night after he had finished the dairy management. The work, of course, caused some noise. One night *ulda-gállis* (the little people's father) came to John Hansen in his dreams and said that he had built the forge upon their home without asking permission. Consequently their children could not fall asleep because of the noise. John Hansen ignored the visit from *ulda-gállis*, but the speaking in his dreams became more frequent. One night he dreamed that *ulda-gállis* was angry and said that if he would not come to an agreement about his work in the forge, he planned to destroy it. John Hansen was frightened and could not continue to behave so rigidly. In the end they agreed that the work should stop by eight o'clock in the evening. After this they lived together in peace.

Ulda is a phenomenon in nature about which the people of the Markebygds learn in early childhood. They learn that nature can be whimsical, and it is best to learn to not ignore omens and other signals. These could be anything from weather prognoses to negotiations with characters. They learn that you have friends in nature if you behave well and loyally. They are faithful that most things can be turned to a good outcome through a form of interaction. In that way, Goffman's concept *order* from 1983 is valid in interactions not only between people but also between people and natural phenomena. Thereby nature is given a state as subject.

Conclusion

The Norwegianization and modernization that came to the Markebygds from the mid-1880s contributed to a change in the way of thinking, which influenced knowledge traditions. As such there was heavy pressure on Sámi culture and language and their ways of practising. The Sámi philosophy of life and cosmologies, as they were expressed through the practices of religion, the practices of Sámi names, and the traditions of healing, was brought into ill repute by various authorities. The same occurred with the arrangements and functioning of everyday life. The *birget* model that searches the repertoire for solutions in the handling of each situation was also discredited. The perpetrators could be teachers, health and agriculture personnel, and gradually also the Laestadian preachers.

The people of the Markebygds placed themselves in negotiation with the actors of the Norwegian systems. We can see in the above accounts that they did not give up all their culture, but sometimes it was necessary to act backstage and, in any case, to go slowly. A consequence of these encounters could be that new experiences gave life to old experiences and led existing phenomena to a new understanding. The intersection of new and old world views yielded insights for a new direction. A new figuration, an innovative process, started. The new situation did not replace the existing one extensively but created an amalgam of both. Thus, new frames that permitted an avoidance of conflicts, on the one hand, had a limiting influence but, on the other hand, facilitated the interaction. We can use the metaphor of building a bridge over troubled water.

For the Markebygd dwellers, their acting together has brought a development of the Markebygd societies and provided opportunities for following new trends. The Markebygds, as shown here, have also welcomed scientific medicine. On this basis they have been able to develop their practices by combining traditions from both folk medicine and scientific medicine. This is illustrated by the keeping of balance, and the keeping of balance was often helped by not being explicit on the thoughts and meanings of the new efforts that were being implemented in the Markebygds. We can conclude that their management of new claims and challenges has been carried out in accordance with Goffman's concepts of playing with the frames (1974), of interaction orders (1983), and of the ongoing presentation of self in everyday life (1992). Each generation, seen from the start of Norwegianization, has its own experiences, and many worthy experiences in their transactions within the local Norwegian arrangements and systems have given good outcomes.

Notes

1. Rossvær's study focuses on a fishing village in Finnmark County. He shows how the fishermen and women adopted the methods of new practices and adapted them to the old practices. In this way, new practices again were created.
2. Christianization of the Sámi started in about the year 1000 with King Olav Tryggvason's journey to the north of Norway to baptize the people. The Sámi mounted a massive resistance (Sturlasson, 1970). It was the beginning of Norwegianization.
3. The primary school law of 1889 for rural areas was signed at Stockholm's Palace, Sweden, on June 26, 1889, to work in conjunction with the primary school law for urban areas. Norway was united with Sweden from May 17, 1814, Norway's Constitution Day, until June 9, 1905 (Norsk utdanningshistorie, https://snl.no/Norsk_utdanningshistorie).
4. In Norway the word *Lapp* is a stigma, a conception for Sámi.
5. A seminar set up by Nordic Sámi Institute Kautokeino at Lavangseidet community house in the municipality of Skånland, in January 2000, in connection with the Norwegian army's plans to place ammunition beside a lake,

Skoddebergvann in Skånland. The intention of the seminar was to present socio-cultural studies, including the history of the area.

6. Aslaug Olsen, who was living in a Markebygd and was interested in kinship relations between Sámi in the north of Sweden and the Markebygds, asked me, when I started my research work, if I knew the story.

References

Aakvaag, G.C. (2008). *Moderne sosiologisk teori* [Modern sociological theory]. Oslo: Abstrakt forlag AS.

Andersen, A. (1999). Minner fra min barndomsskolegang på Boltås skole [Memories from my childhood school time at the School of Boltås]. *Debattsiden, Harstad Tidende* [The Page of Discussion, Newspaper of Harstad], August 10.

Bateson, G. (1973). *Steps to an ecology of mind*. St. Albans, UK: Paladin.

Berkes, F., Colding, J., & Folke, C. (2000). Rediscovery of traditional ecological knowledge as adaptive management. *Ecological Applications by the Ecological Society of America, 10*(5), 1251–1262.

Christensen, O. (1997). Diskriminering og rasisme [Discrimination and racism]. In T.H. Eriksen (Ed.), *Flerkulturell forståelse* [Multicultural understanding] (pp. 90–107). Oslo: Tano Aschehoug.

Drivenes, E.-A., Hauan, M.A., & Wold, H.A. (Eds.). (1994). *Nordnorsk kulturhistorie: Det gjenstridige landet* [The cultural history of North Norway: The obstinate land]. Oslo: Gyldendal Norsk Forlag.

Dunfjeld, M. (2006). *Tjaalehtjimmie: Form og innhold i sørsamisk ornamentikk* [Form and content in south Sámi ornamentation]. Snåsa, Norway: Saemien Sijte.

Foley, D. (2005). Indigenous standpoint theory: An acceptable academic process for indigenous academics. (Melbourne, Australia). *International Journal of the Humanities, 3*(8), 25–36.

Foss, C., & Eilifsen, B. (2004). De utydelige overtramp? Etiske utfordringer ved kvalitative studier [The unclear violations? Ethical challenges with qualitative studies]. *Vård i Norden* [Nursing Science and Research in the Nordic Countries], 24(3), 48–51.

Goffman, E. (1974). *Frame analysis: An essay on the organization of experience*. New York: Harper.

Goffman, E. (1983). The Interaction Order. *American Sociological Review, 4*(8), 1–17.

Goffman, E. (1992). *Vårt rollespill til daglig: En studie i hverdagslivets dramatikk* [The presentation of self in everyday life, 1959]. Oslo: Pax Forlag A/S.

Helander, E. (2004). *Samiska rättsuppfattningar* [Sámi understandings of law]. Rovaniemi, Finland: Juridica Lapponica 30 Oy Sevenprint Ltd.

Helander-Renvall, E. (2008). Animism, personhood, and the nature of reality: Sami perspectives. *Polar Record, 46*(236), 44–56.

Kalstad, J.K.H. (1997). Reindriftspolitikk og samisk kultur—en uløselig konflikt? En studie av reindriftstilpasninger og moderne reindriftspolitikk [The policy of reindeer husbandry and Sámi culture—an unsolvable conflict? A study of adaptions of reindeer husbandry and modern policy of reindeer husbandry]. Doctoral dissertation, Universitetet i Tromsø.

Kleinman, A. (1980). *Patient and healers in context of culture: An exploration of the borderland between anthropology, medicine, and psychiatry.* London: University of California Press.

Løken, O. (1900). Distriktslæge i Skjervø. In *Beretning om Sundhedstilstanden og Medicinalforholdene i Norge 1900* [Physician of District of Skjervø. In *Report about the state of health and the conditions of medicine in Norway, 1900*]. Norges officielle Statistikk [The official statistics of Norway]. Fjerde Række Nr.55 Udgiven af Direktøren for det civile Medicinalvæsen. Kristiania (Oslo): I kommisjon hos H. Aschehoug.

Mathisen, S.R. (1989). Den etniske grensen mellom nordmenn og samer [The ethnical border between Norwegians and Sámi]. *Norveg: Folkelivsgransking, 32*, 105–115.

Mathisen, S.R. (2000). Folkemedisinen i Nord-Norge: Kulturelt fellesskap og etniske skillelinjer [Folk medicine in North Norway: Cultural fellowship and ethnic divisions]. In I. Altern & G.-T. Minde (Eds.), *Samisk folkemedisin i dagens Norge* [Sámi folk medicine in today's Norway] (pp. 15–33). Tromsø: Universitetet i Tromsø, Senter for samiske studier / Sámi dutkamiid guovddás.

Minde, H. (1997). *Diktning og historie om samene på Stuoranjarga, Rapport II: Skoddebergprosjektet* [Writing and history about the Sámi at Stuoranjarga (Skånland and Evenes), Report 2: The project of Skoddeberg]. Tromsø: Universitetet i Tromsø, Sámi Instituhtta / Sámi dutkamiid guovddaš.

Nakata, M. (2007). *Disciplining the savages. Savaging the disciplines.* Canberra: Aboriginal Studies Press.

NOU (Norges offentlige utredninger, Norwegian Official Report). (1995). *Plan for helse- og sosialtjenester til den samiske befolkning i Norge* [Plan of health and social services for the Sámi population in Norway]. Oslo: Statens Forvaltningstjeneste.

Nymo, R. (2003). *"Har løst å kle på sæ kofte, men tør ikkje og vil ikkje": En studie av fornorskning, identitet og kropp blant samer i Ofoten og Sør-Troms* ["I'd like to wear my national costume, but I daren't and won't": A study of Norwegianization, identity and body among Sámi in Ofoten and southern Troms]. Master's thesis, University of Tromsø, Hovedfagsoppgave i helsefag.

Nymo, R. (2011). Helseomsorgssystemer i de samiske markebygder i Nordre Nordland og Sør-Troms: Praksiser i hverdagslivet; "En ska ikkje gje sæ over og en ska ta tida til hjelp" [Health-care systems in Sámi woodland parishes of northern Nordland County and southern Troms County: Everyday life practices; "One should not succumb and one should take time as an aid"]. Doctoral dissertation, University of Tromsø, Faculty of Health Science, Department of Health and Caring.

Osgood, J. (2010). Narrative methods in the nursery: (Re)considering claims to give voice through processes of decision-making. *Reconceptualizing Educational Research Methodology (RERM)*, 1, 14–28.

Oslo kommune [Oslo municipality]. (1932). Fra varm mat til oslofrokost til matpakke [From warm food to Oslo breakfast to lunch packet]. http://www.byarkivet.oslo. kommune.no/OBA/Mat/oslofrokost.asp

Porsanger, J. (2004). An essay about indigenous methodology. *Nordlit, Special Issue on Northern Minorities*, 15, 105–120.

Porsanger, J. (2010). Self-determination and indigenous research: Capacity building on our own terms. In V. Tauli-Corpuz, L. Enkiwe-Abayao, & R. de Chavez (Eds.), *Towards an alternative development paradigm: Indigenous peoples' self-determined development* (pp. 433–446). Baguio City, Philippines: Tebtebba Foundation.

Rolf, B. (1995). *Profession, Tradition och tyst kunskap En studie i Michael Polanyis teori om den professionella kunskapens tysta dimension* [Profession, tradition, and tacit knowledge: A study in Michael Polanyi's theory about the professional knowledge's tacit dimension]. Övre Dalskarlshyttan, Sweden: Bokförlaget Nya Doxa AB.

Rossvær, V. (1998). *Ruinlandskap og modernitet* [Ruined landscape and modernity]. Oslo: Spartacus Forlag.

Smith, L.T. (1999). *Decolonizing methodologies: Research and indigenous peoples.* London: Zed Books, University of Otago Press.

Sturlasson, S. (1970). *Snorres kongesagaer: Heimskringla* [The kings' sagas of Snorre]. Oslo: Gyldendal Norsk Forlag.

Thorne, S. (1993). Secondary analysis in qualitative research: Issues and implications. In J.M. Morse (Ed.), *Critical issues in qualitative research methods* (pp. 263–279). Thousand Oaks, CA: Sage.

Van Manen, M. (2007). *Researching, lived experience human science for an action sensitive pedagogy.* Winnipeg, MB: Althouse Press.

Verran, H. (2005). Knowledge traditions of aboriginal Australians: Questions and answers arising in a databasing project. http://www.cdu.edu.au/centres/ik/pdf/ knowledgeanddatabasing.pdf.

Wicklund, L. (2008). Patient perspectives: Existential aspects of living with addiction; Part I, Meeting challenges. *Journal of Clinical Nursing, 17*, 2426–2434.

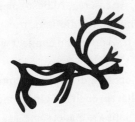

Gifts of Dreams
Connecting to Sámi Epistemic Practice

BRITT KRAMVIG

This chapter explores dreaming and gift giving to see their connection to
Sámi epistemic practice and knowledge traditions. In the Coastal Sámi
communities where I have been doing fieldwork, dreams are part of the
local practices. In addition, the Sámi language is rarely used in everyday
life. The particular colonial history in many northern communities of
Sápmi has implied that Sáminess has become complex and ambiguous.
Identities are fluid where places, families, and personal stories often
become assemblages of the three different ethnic groups—Norwegian,
Sami, and Kvæn—that for centuries have settled on the Sámi people's traditional land. Locally, people talk about themselves as being a mixture of different historical puzzles and heterogeneous relationships, as well as taking
part in ongoing negotiations. Even though the Sámi language has been
lost for many people, spiritual knowledge traditions are still vivid, at least
for some. This paves the way for highly heterogeneous ideas about spiritual matters. People insist on multiplicity and ambiguity when it comes to

articulating spirituality. Spirituality reconnects to the Sámi heritage, with its concern for the future, the capacity to make better decisions, and the performance of colonial resistance. It is multiple and ambiguous. Inspired by the post-colonial writer Spivak (1985/1994), we can regard post-colonial identities as the outcome of a network of multiple contradictions, traces, and inscriptions, which are still struggling to hold on to and connect with Sámi knowledge traditions.

In the first section of this chapter I will explore how dreaming becomes part of reconnecting. In addition, I will argue that through the gift, or more precisely through giving, relations and connections are made; some, as Mauss (1970) argues, ask for a gift in return, and in others, giving is performing the person's relationships, network, and identities in relationship to others. I will argue that via dreaming, the spiritual life of people, animals, and nature comes into reality. What becomes real, within what I will call upon as Sámi epistemic practice, needs to be revisited. The reconnections that are accomplished through dreaming, and the influence that the dreams have, is a highly flexible matter. It is considered to be the dreamer's responsibility to do the interpretative work; dreams fuel and work side by side with other practices that foreshadow the autonomy of the person (Kramvig, 2005). The autonomy of the person is highly prized in these societies where people live in relation to one another and are still dependent upon nature and natural resources. It goes with the capacity to make relevant decisions in relation to rapid, and often violent, changes in the weather conditions in an arctic environment; people take pride in having the capacity to manage "on their own," living in what other people consider to be the margins. I will also ask, however, whether autonomy becomes something that is even more important to handle with tenderness and care in indigenous communities where decolonization is an ongoing situation, where the presence of the colonial Other within the self is a blurred and often shameful presence, and where these contradictions are mostly silenced in the public debate. Western scientific epistemology is enacted to keep categories clean and in place, and distinctions are made between real and unreal, the natural and the supernatural, culture and nature. Sámi epistemic practice reconnects to the past and future whereby community is formed.

I will argue that the dreaming enacts and performs collective memories. It is a practice (or at least it contains the traces of a practice) in the here and now, in which is found reconnection to the indigenous past. It involves mimesis. Dreams, at the same time, pave the way for a more concerned and conscious approach to the ongoing life and the challenges that people face, for example, when it comes to the matter of life and death. My theoretical concerns relate to what dreams do, and by that I will insist upon considering them as relational, which is more than what appearance would concede.

The concept of mimesis needs some clarification. Mimesis is seen, inspired by Taussig (1993), Stoller (1995), and Willerslev (2007), as both copying the colonial and having sensuous contact with the collective memories. Mimesis relates to copying the colonial Other and, by doing so, creating a ground for awareness of the presence of the Other in the self, but still maintaining and creating a sensuous contact with the indigenous knowledge traditions. Mimesis can work through dreaming and by telling people about the dreams. Dreaming secures a sense of autonomy, wherein telling people about the dream secures the social aspect and works on remodelling the indigenous community in which these practices belong. It becomes, as Helen Verran (2004) argues, an alternative way of managing contradiction and points to "a blind-spot embedded in the Western cultural unconscious, yet which is significant for postcolonial critique" (p. 149).

The Legacy of Colonialism

The legacy of colonialism includes the subjugation and marginalization of indigenous people's ways and practices of knowing; this knowing comprehends the honouring of the subtle and vital connections between the natural environment, people, and other living beings. Recently, decennia after overt colonialism, some adjustments in the legacy of colonialism have been made; Norway adopted a Sámi law in 1987, amended its constitution in 1988, and ratified International Labour Organization (ILO) Convention 169, which concerned indigenous and tribal people in 1990, binding the government to practise its legislation in accordance with international law (Minde, 2008). The opening of the Sámi parliament in Norway, Sámediggi, in 1989 was a turning point in the political scene. It was followed by a land-reform process that was initiated by the transfer of 45,000 square kilometres of state land to a non-governmental body, Finnmark Estate, in 2006, fuelling the decolonization processes that may be observed in contemporary society. This can be seen as a process that is moving away from an old "frontier order" of the North that is dominated by the nation-state towards a new social order, a "homeland" situation providing northern citizens with increasing self-governing capacity and the potential for improved welfare and progress (Sandberg, 2009). There are several unsolved issues in regard to land claims (and a very intense local debate), which involve new systems of government and the production of new management regimes in Sápmi. Despite these positive developments, colonial dynamics continue to influence Sámi communities via ongoing governmental institutions and policies and through the new industrial turn in the Arctic; they also continue in the more informal and multi-faceted processes of community and autonomy. These dynamics still hinder the process toward full recognition of the right to self-determination, which parallels the quest for the recognition of indigenous knowledge. Watson-Verran and Turnbull (1995) argue against the marginalization of indigenous knowledge, and they also note a distinct cultural bias in its evaluation:

> By and large, past cross-cultural work has taken Western "rationality" and "scientificity" as the benchmark criteria by which other cultures' knowledge should be evaluated. So-called traditional knowledge systems of indigenous peoples have frequently been portrayed as closed, pragmatic, utilitarian, value-laden, indexical, context-dependent, and so on, implying that they cannot have the same authority and credibility as science because their localness restricts them to the social and cultural circumstances of their production. (pp. 115–116)

The epistemic encompasses knowing as practice. This is an argument to the effect that indigenous ways of knowing are equally valid as tools, not only for understanding the local conditions of existence but also for providing knowledge of great interest to the wider scientific community (Kuokkanen, 2007). The Sámi scholar Rauna Kuokkanen (2010, p. 75) conceptualizes indigenous world views in terms of the "indigenous episteme": "I employ the concept of 'episteme' to denote ways of knowing, understanding and relating to the world. Referring to worldviews or ontologies, episteme is, therefore, a broader concept than epistemology."

Indigenous people's claims to land rights are based on the notion that they have a relationship with the territories that they have historically inhabited and continue to inhabit. In an indigenous context, efforts toward formulating rights to land and water and other cultural rights are often grounded in the view that people and nature are interrelated. Though the colonial situation has served to sever these bonds, it is still seen, at least for some, as vital for the well-being of people and the natural environment to restore the resulting imbalances. This understanding of nature, or world view, does not imply a return to pre-colonial realities; it expresses an epistemic culture that is adequate to face the challenges of modern times. If not a return to, it does mean a re-connection with the past in order for traditional forms of knowledge, and ways of being in the world, to continue to be expressed in modern-day society.

Political autonomy, as argued by Sámi political bodies, is advanced by the continuing decolonization politics. Even so, the way in which autonomies are handled in everyday life in these communities needs to be approached because it plays a part in the way in which autonomy should be handled in political discourses and white papers. Within the Sámi communities (as in other Western communities), autonomy is of utmost importance, yet there are differences that need to be articulated. I will take up these arguments by addressing the "performativity" of the gift and showing that it has the capacity to establish flexible and fluid communities while performing indigenous resistance and autonomy.

I have been living in and have travelled in and out of different municipalities in Finnmark County for two decades now. On the move, like others in this Arctic sea- and landscape, yet still trained within anthropology, I wanted to carry out "proper" ethnographic fieldwork in one of the Coastal Sámi communities for my doctorate. What I learned from people who generously set out to "teach the student" was, in my mind, as important as what I learned from the books I have read and the life I have lived. Ingmar, an old fisherman and one of the few locals still speaking Sámi, was one of those who first took me into their life, home, and way of life. Like others in his community, he also moved in and out of this remote (in regard to public transportation) yet still vibrant fishing village, a village in which people came together in community, fighting to survive at a time that most other villages on the coast of Finnmark were suffering from dramatic population declines. Ingmar is our guide to Sámi dreaming epistemology.

Dreaming and Mimesis

Ingmar was born into a Coastal Sámi community in the beginning of the twentieth century. Early in his life Ingmar (who appears in many of my ethnographic texts—2003, 2005, 2009) had dreams of great importance to him: "I was 19 the first time I was in mortal danger. Then I dreamed that I was walking across a bridge, and the bridge was an arch like a rainbow. The bridge got narrower and narrower, and I thought to myself, 'This isn't the track I'm supposed to follow.' Then I managed to turn around. And when I'd managed to turn, I could go back. And when I woke up, I felt much better."

The dream provided insight that Ingmar could use to rid himself of what was ailing him. Dreaming created a reality of othering, and, through this othering, a reconnection could be made. It made way for redoing the presence of the colonial Other in the self. Paying attention to the dream is in itself a reconnecting to the Sámi epistemic practice. In the dream Ingmar experiences "I could go back." The "going back" in the present is a recalling of the new tracks that he himself should follow for the rest of his life. Through his following of these other tracks and managing to turn back, and by his listening and acting within a specific epistemic practice, a situation appeared that also had the capacity to bring about the healing process through which he himself became redone as a person. For Ingmar, dreams are not seen as outside the circumstances of the ordinary; they are a way of seeing. We can note that in this practice of dreaming there is the possibility of othering, and, by that, of seeing the autonomy and possibility of the individual Sámi self. By having the insight into the dream, Ingmar made a connection, and he could make better decisions in relation to the challenges that appeared as important along the journey of life. This is a form of mimesis, one in which Ingmar could communicate with himself about his life, and which provided the opportunity to acquire insight into the foundation of his own life as well as the lives of others.

I have found few references to dreams in the literature about the Sámi world, and even fewer in studies about the northern regions. An exception is Knut Odner's (1995) article on Sámi identity, which contains accounts of several dreams. Odner maintains that many inhabitants of Lakseby regard dreams as social facts or what he calls "condensed reality" (p. 135). This is not a bad term. "Condensed consciousness," he says, "removes the boundaries between realities. You are torn out of the semi-lethargic reality which is earthly real and transported into another reality in which ordinary sensory and physical limitations no longer exist" (ibid.). I am not sure that Ingmar was torn out of our ordinary sensory worlds in his dreams. I think, rather, that these dreams, in all their richness, offer an opportunity for insight into the reality of the everyday. These in turn offer the ability to change tracks in life. Bente Alver (1997) makes a similar reflection in her description of an encounter with the Sámi woman Mari. Mari was ill and wanted to tell Alver about her life in order to understand it better herself. She talked about one of the many dreams that she described as being turning points in her life. For three nights in a row Mari dreamed that her paternal grandmother asked her to put flowers on her grave. After consulting her father, Mari realized that she had to make this journey in her dream, which she did the next time the dream occurred. But she was led astray and did not find the grave until a bird assisted her. Mari saw this both as a test of whether she was brave enough to visit the land of the dead and as a test of her patience and obedience (Alver, 1997, pp. 114–115).

There is some resonance between Ingmar's and Mari's stories. Both Ingmar and Mari saw their dreams as offering important guidelines for their own lives. They both were tested and had to be able to "grasp" and act upon the challenges presented by the dreams. The dreams were turning points in their lives through which they were given insight that they had not had before. For Ingmar, the dream also brought healing, which is not highlighted by Alver for Mari; however, there is a need expressed, and then a method for improving the situation.

Kapferer (1997) has argued that it is necessary to look at dreams and forms of healing as ingredients of everyday life. Dreams give direction to life, and as the life differs, so they differ radically from one part of the world to another (ibid.). They are not models for or of reality but instead constitute realities in themselves that have to be seen in relation to the people as well as the landscape, from which they appear and to which they communicate. For Ingmar, it was important to be able to hear what the dream told him and to be able to act, both in the dream and afterwards, in accordance with the dream. Ingmar said that when he dreamed about women and halibut, all he had to do was to take his boat out and pull up the seine that he had cast, and then he would usually have a large catch. The dreaming of halibut and women gave direction to the fisherman, but it had to be acted upon. Dreams, Kapferer says, are not primarily fantasies, nor are they outside the actualities of the lived world. Dreams are "like acts of the imagination of consciousness, resulting from the dwelling of human beings in the world, no matter how" (ibid., p. 180).

Mimetic Faculty as Part of Decolonization

Taussig (1993) calls upon the concept of mimetic faculty as the nature that culture uses to create second nature and as the faculty to cope, imitate, make models, explore difference, and yield into and become Other. It is a two-way street, whereby histories enter into the functioning of the mimetic faculty, and the mimetic faculty enters into those histories. In some way, one can protect oneself from the Other by portraying them. "Pulling you this way and that, mimesis plays this trick of dancing between the very same and the very different. An impossible but necessary, indeed an every-day affair, mimesis registers both sameness and difference, of being like, and of being Other" (Taussig, 1993, p. 129).

Dreaming can be seen as the part in between. In Sámi the concept of *adjagas* relates to this moment of being and not being awake at the same time. It is a tender moment and is still full of potential. In *adjagas*, recon-nection with the Sámi landscape, ancestors, and spirits can come into being (Gaski, 2008). Stories, images, or a *joik* coming from a specific place appear to the person in the moment between sleep and awakening. By the performance of memories and stories from a specific place to a person, that person is connected or reconnected to the landscape or the past. An example can be given. When I got married, the ritual was held in a cave (named Kirkhelleren) on one of the many islands on the coast of Helgeland in Northern Norway. This is an area were local historians and local mimesis emphasize the cultural heritage as being Norwegian, although this view can be contested; archaeology and history tell a different and more complex story of the dynamic migration of Sámi and Norwegian settlements in the area. One of our friends attending the wedding was a young Sámi artist, and he was going to the cave for the first time. One night prior to arriving he had a dream in which he found himself in the cave. Dwelling within that landscape, a *joik* came before him. It was the voice of the place, the sense of the place, that came in the dream. He awoke with the *joik* still present. Kirkhelleren was announcing itself as real and came into the life of the person through the dream. When the artist arrived, he brought this *joik* and performed it in our wedding cave. Therefore, the *joik* of the cave came back to the cave, and this reconnection brought the Sámi heritage into the present and into real existence, a presence that had been forgotten for a long time. After the event some of the people from the area came to him, fumbling but still talking about the sorrow of their own loss of connection with Sámi heritage, a heritage almost forgotten but one that was recalled by the event.

Adjagas, the "between," can be found elsewhere, as in Moroccan mystical thinking. In the book *Imaginative Horizons*, Crapanzano (2003) describes the way in which Abedsalem, his Moroccan friend and mentor, thought of the between. For Abedsalem, the between is "*barzakh*," and *barzakh* is what lies between things—between edges, borders, and events. He likened it to the silence between words and dreams. "The dream is between waking life and sleep." The notion of the between has deep roots in Sufi thought. In the mystical world of the Sufi philosopher al-Arabi, the imagination, like the between and the state of disease remission, is indeterminate. At times it appears to be between the spiritual and the material (the sensuous) world. At others, between being and nothingness is somehow equivalent to existence. Crapanzano (2003) argues that the important point is that the imagination is an intermediate "reality," inherently ambiguous, and best described as "neither this nor that, or both this and that."

Put another way, the imaginative interstices of the between become, for many of us, spaces of ambiguity that can generate fear and anxiety. And yet, dwelling in the between can also be illuminating. Crapanzano (2003) points out that the liminal has often been likened to the dream. It suggests imaginative possibilities that are not necessarily available to us in everyday life.

Through paradox, ambiguity, and contradiction and the evocation of transcendent realities, mystery, and supernatural powers, the liminal offers us a view of the world to which we are normally blinded by the usual structures of social and cultural life. The liminal therefore can be a space of creative imagination, of provocative linkages, and of personal empowerment.

Dwelling with Ingmar and others within the community where I did fieldwork meant that I was present when the dreaming was discussed on different important occasions. Following are three examples. In one episode, the Sámi herder Per, who lived in one of the villages during the summer and herded reindeer, was lost at sea. It had been a nice early-summer's day when Per had taken the boat out fishing. He was on his own, and some said it had also been "a long night." Some hours later, they found the boat empty and started searching for Per. A member of the emergency coast guard was called upon, but he was out on some other duty. That night, the young herder Johan had a dream in which Per came to him and gave him the direction to where he could be found. The coast guard came the next morning, and the direction was given to him. The coast guard followed these directions, and soon afterwards Per's body was found in open waters.

In another example, one early morning a young, local fisherman, Jens, was walking the shoreline of the island where he lived. People used to do that occasionally after stormy weather because it brought different and sometimes valuable items onto the shore. Jens said he saw the skin of a reindeer, but, upon coming closer, he saw that this was a body that had been brought in by the sea, having stayed in open water for some time. He was quite shaken and called the police. He could not rest until they had come and removed the body. Later, during an interview by the local newspaper *Finnmark dagblad*,[1] he expressed the surprise that he had felt upon learning the name of the person he had found. Some nights prior to finding the body, Jen had dreamed that the perished fisherman had approached him, telling him his name and that he had been fishing and had fallen overboard. The perished fisherman was not local, so people did not know him well. Jens did not remember his full name when he awoke, but he remembered the letter *E* or *G*. He told his friends, and then, when the name was actually known and indeed had the sounds of *E* and *G* in it, his dream information was confirmed. He did not have the sense that the dream was a nightmare; on the contrary, it was the fisherman who had needed to explain who he was and where he could be found. He had expressed his gratitude toward Jens in that dream, and therefore the dream appeared to Jens as something good.

Another example was told when I was out fishing with a local woman, Inga. She pointed to the place where one of her relatives had been surprised by bad weather and where the empty boat had been found. Inga said that they set out to search for him and after some days decided that if he were not found alive, they would still search for him to give him a grave. Months later he appeared in a dream of Inga, telling her that he was safe and calm and that there was no need to search for him any longer, that he had found his grave.

The psychology of dreaming has received varying interpretations. Freud and Oppenheim (1958) looked at dreams as the manifestation of the unconscious, in which were pictured those instinctual drives and desires that we needed to repress in our everyday waking life; in this way, Freud claimed, dreams gave us a guideline to how the unconscious worked. This differs from the way in which dreams are interpreted in my community: dreaming directs the attention of the dreamer; it is for the dreamer to pay attention to and reflect upon the stories told in the dream. The interpretation is not scripted or made by others; it is for the dreamer to make sense of it. The dreamer's interpretation depends upon the life into which the dream fits. Some would say that you should not tell anybody about the dream, because therefore it would not be fulfilled. Others find it acceptable to tell people about the dream, as we see in Jens's relating of his dream to the newspaper. Dreams, as we have seen about the lost fishermen, make connections. These dreams give consolation and reconciliation to those in need of it. What I hope to have highlighted is that, through dreams, a connection to past events and an influence on the future were achieved.

The interpretation of dreams by Freud and as understood in Sápmi, where I reside, relate to different ontological assumptions and different epistemic practices. The dreamer in Sápmi engages himself in or with the world, independent of whether he is asleep or awake. There is no conflict between the dream and the awake state; moreover, during dreaming, the spirituality becomes somewhat real, and as a result it can heal relationships and the bodies of those present, as happened with the body of Ingmar when he followed the direction presented to him by the dream. Similarly, Willerslev's (2007) ethnography draws upon fieldwork among the Siberian Yukaghirs, and it is argued that dreams are understood as "doing" and that they are part of both the conscious and the self-conscious or reflexive life (p. 178). For Yukaghirs, dream imagery reflects the experience of the soul, which is considered capable of influencing events, giving personal advantage through sexual engagement with spiritual beings. Contrasting Freud, Willerslev states: "Freud, like many other Western thinkers, starts with the premise that the mind is distinct from the world, which is why dreams, in his theory, only reflect one's inner state. For Yukaghirs, on the contrary, the mind always subsists in the very engagement of the person in the world, quite independently of whether he is asleep or awake" (p. 176). He suggests that regardless of whether one is awake or asleep, the personal encounters are always those of being in a world—and never an "empty reality," as suggested by Freud. Secondly, the awareness of the dreaming self is as phenomenally real as when a person is awake (Willerslev, 2007, p. 178).

The healing tradition is part and parcel of the Sámi world view or tradition of knowing (Kramvig, 2003; Miller, 2007; Myrvoll, 2010), and I will argue that dreaming is too. In practice, what this means is that one works with the kinds of challenges that are so often carried out by individuals alone, and then transfers this to a collective level (to look at it from a distance) where the individual is relieved of the sole responsibility of processing the grief, frustrations, and shame that the living of colonized lives implies. As such, the indigenous episteme is expressed in the everyday work of remembering and articulating the old ways in forms that communicate with present-day Sámi and colonial realities, thereby instigating the healing of deep colonial wounds. With Butler (2003), we can say that the mourning of loss defies nostalgia and instead implies the forming of an "active and open relationship to history," a creative practice in which the pain that could not be lived fully in the past is in fact lived and released in the present. Working with such processes at a community level, "loss becomes a condition and necessity for a certain sense of community...the pathos is not negated, but it turns out to be oddly fecund, paradoxically productive" (Butler, 2003, p. 468).

The Gift as an Expression of Sámi Epistemic Practices

Dreaming is performative; it is part of the reconnections made in the everyday. The dreaming practice is related to acts of giving; it is a practice that recalls the interconnectedness of people, nature, and landscape. In previous publications (Kramvig, 2005, 2009) I have argued that the autonomy and community that traffic ethnic boundaries are expressed through the process of giving. This means that gift giving implies the potential for breaking with the more static understandings of identities, communities, and the relationship between nature and culture; therefore, by using the notion of the gift as an ontological starting point and considering community as performed in the here and now (Verran, 2002), we follow a performance that can be found by following the gift.

Marcel Mauss's (1990) influential essay on the gift has been an inspiration for theorizing the gift in a vast range of studies, including both feminist and indigenous studies. The gift concerns not only the exchange of material objects but also the flow of social and cultural relations. It comes with a magical power that forces the gift to circulate and return, or, as Mauss puts it, "a gift is received 'with a burden attached'" (1990, p. 41). Specifically, the gift in Sápmi implies a performance of wide networks of relationships that are both concrete and subtle (Kramvig, 2009). The logic of the gift challenges, and sometimes subverts, the logic of the market economy, stressing the circulation of objects in the subsistence sphere, but it also has a far wider significance. It is a notion that expresses both the cultural and the natural aspects of interrelatedness.

Gifts in Sápmi come in many shapes, but often as food. Food is not given to just anyone; gifts of food flow within a network of individuals who, in various ways and to varying degrees, are dependent on one another. These gifts relate to the history of these individuals' significance to each other; even the gifts tell them who they are. In the summer, when the fisherman brings in the boat after fishing for pollock, the day's catch is shared among some but not all of those present on the quay. The meaning of social relations can be mapped by following the sharing of fish, fish cakes, and woollen socks. Identities are performed through these gifts. Through the process of gift giving, people's individuality and sense of self are fortified, and at the same moment connections to others are made. The processes promote and reaffirm not only individual autonomy but also a sense of community. Through these gifts the possibility of drawing a locally applicable distinction between themselves and others appears. Equality based on the gift as a mechanism of social inclusion give rise to a network of interrelated people, and several networks arise in the locality involving people from the local community and relatives and friends from further away—in the region or country as a whole and even abroad.

In indigenous feminist writing, these aspects of the gift have been taken further: "The purpose of giving...is to acknowledge and renew the sense of kinship and co-existence with the world. In other words, the gift is the manifestation of reciprocity with one's ecosystem, reflecting the bond of dependence and respect towards the natural world. From this bond, certain responsibilities emerge" (Kuokkanen, 2006, p. 13).

Becoming Kin, Becoming Sámi

The Sámi gift-exchange systems have a kind of openness that allows people to enter them without being seen as the same as others. Equality created by the gift tends to be seen as more important than the equality viewed as sameness. The gift makes it possible for strangers to be integrated and positioned in the local contexts, despite any differences the stranger might exhibit. I argue below for an articulation of the gift-exchange mechanism in the context of Sámi kinship systems. Pehrson's (1964) *Bilateral Network of Social Relations in the Könkämä Lapp District* is one early ethnographic study carried out on Sámi kinship. His main argument is that Sámi kinship is bilateral and that kinship structure determines most other social relations. "The Lappish mode of reckoning kinship and of transmitting property is also the Lappish mode of selecting leaders, structuring relationship termin-ology and providing the individual with work mates, trading partners and band fellows" (p. 107). Flexibility, variability, and a lack of corporate groups are some of those elements that he sees as being characteristic of the Sámi social system. This flexibility can be seen in the *verddet* institution.

The Sámi *verddet* is a community, partly kinship based, partly social, securing relationships within the different areas that herders will traverse in the year cycle. At the same time, it is involved in gift giving, where items and services circulate (Bjørklund & Eidheim, 1999). *Verddet* has also played an essential role in ensuring sufficient manpower for the reindeer *siidas* during both the herding and the sedentary seasons. The *siida* is a local Sámi community that has existed from time immemorial. The reindeer-herding *siida* has adapted ancient *siida* principles to large-scale nomadic reindeer herding. It is a basic organizational unit for carrying out large-scale herding, which was not legally acknowledged by the Norwegian national authorities until recently (Sara, 2009). Another important aspect of the community is the knowledge embedded in the *siida's* practices and everyday dealings with the local environment. The use of traditional Sámi reindeer-herding practices and knowledge is closely related to the viability of the *siida* system (ibid.). It is a highly flexible system (as is the *verddet*) for securing sufficient manpower for the task at hand. During the spring the reindeer are moved from their winter pastures on the mainland to the summer pastures on the coast; the most labour-intensive stages involve moving the herd in and out of the area that is reserved for earmarking the calves, transportation to and from the island, and slaughtering. Obviously sufficient manpower is essential, and labour tends to come from the family, partial owners of the herd, and people from where the herd is stationed during the season. These are long-term relationships that can be activated and even transmitted down through the generations. The help given can be compensated by reindeer produce or other services considered as reasonable by convention. Money seldom figures, if ever, in these transactions. The people involved often refer to each other with the term *verdde*. This *verddet* institution can be activated in any of the districts through which the animals pass during the course of the year. Some of the reindeer in the herd used to be *verddet* owned, and these are given their own special earmark (Bjørklund & Eidheim, 1999).

That kinship has been the most important organizational category of Sámi society, and at the same time the Sámi kinship classification system is distinguished by its openness, and the willingness to integrate others is a paradox that most Sámi studies have generally ignored.

Despite the assimilation policies affecting the local knowledge traditions (in these multi-ethnic communities), Finnish and Norwegian immigrants were integrated into the existing social fabric through intermarriage or by inclusion in the gift system. Pehrson (1964) argues that continuity in Sámi social structure cannot be traced in the stable maintenance of the community but rather in the types of relationships that have prevailed. Such performative systems are in constant flux, but nevertheless they retain their core integrative function. In order to gain acceptance in the community, one has to assume a place in the gift-exchange system. Now, as Hoem (1999) argues, the performative structure may be applicable to the Sámi way of organizing their social system. The performative structures found today are not specifically Sámi, Norwegian, or Finnish, of course, but inasmuch as they work to strengthen ethnic integration, they can be said to be strongly co-extensive with historical Sámi social structures. At the same time, the gift becomes a way of dramatizing these other group boundaries or lines. In general, recognition can be achieved by two different means: either by forcing people to acknowledge recognition by mastering them, or by receiving recognition as a gift from others, signifying a desire for mutual recognition. Therefore, power can be an element of recognition. However, the recognition of which Ricoeur (2005) speaks, and which the silent language of the gift can create, can be seen as a community-forming practice. The kind of reciprocity that involves recognition can be experienced through the mutual recognition that comes with the gift. The meaning of the gift is a question that must be raised within the context in which the gift is given, and it may turn out to have several shades of meaning, as I have tried to illustrate.

Gift as Mutual Recognition and Resistance

The gift economy in Sápmi can be seen as a form of cultural resistance against the logic of Others. The Others in this setting, as is often the case, is a vague category that varies according to context. The praxis of gift-giving systems and a gift economy ritualize those values that have importance in the community, and I have argued that gift giving is important in the creation both of individual autonomy and of community and can be recognized in the Sámi *verddet* institution and symbolic kinship relation. Both the Sami *verddet* institution and the symbolic kinship relation have the capacity to integrate differences through the symbolic relationships created in these institutions. A sense of community that can exceed ethnic and other differences is created in these processes, thereby setting up boundaries and creating community by other means than the conventional categories of ethnicity, class, and gender.

Kuokkanen (2006) argues that the gift paradigm represents a radical challenge to the dominant market liberalism, and for that reason it should be considered a model of differences and one that can show how women's autonomy is emerging in post-colonial indigenous societies. An example can be helpful. After several years, Eline (the woman with whom I used to stay during my ethnographic work in one of the communities) told me that she had enrolled in the Sámi parliament election register a few years ago in order to have the right to vote, but that she "did not like to brag about it." For her, ethnicity was enacted in the practices for which Sámi women like herself gained respect from others within her local community. This respect was not expected from the society as a whole, she knew. "They consider us to be 'Finn' out here, and for that reason we are not as highly respected as Norwegians," she would say, but even so she kept to her own way of being and doing. Her way of tackling the world in which she lived was local and mostly subsistent. However, the gift economy is addressed in a global indigenous field as well as the feminist research field (Kuokkanen, 2006), and by this she can enter into a position where her way of doing becomes recognized outside of the local and everyday practices. The post-colonial in this sense becomes the local resistance against the dominant market liberalism, and the insistence upon the gift is the local, ecological, and persistent economy, as well as being an epistemic practice. Therefore, by this movement Eline appears as a Sámi and an indigenous woman, and by this movement she is given recognition and autonomy even within a global discourse on indigenousness.

When Dreaming Becomes Part of the Ethnographic Work

The ethnographer is in a position to learn, but how does this come about? When science is considered a knowledge system alongside indigenous knowledge systems (Watson-Verran & Turnbull, 1995)—or is seen as different knowledge traditions (as the concept was later developed by Verran, 2002)—how are we to articulate ethnographic work? First of all, when we do ethnography, we also do theory. We bring issues and predications, visions, specific questions, and sensibilities into the field and into our academic office, and those materials reflect, embed, disturb, and perform preoccupations. The post-colonial literature reminds us that there is much at stake when dominant and subaltern knowledge traditions encounter each other.

Law and Lin (2011) argue that the Western legacy carries and reproduces a specific form of metaphysics, it rests on and stabilizes around some specific institutional arrangements, and these imply particular subjectivities. We used to talk about the empirical and the theoretical and the way the theoretical reworked the empirical. One of the post-colonial suggestions is to let this distinction go. Another way is to consider these as two different metaphysical ideas, distinct and different ways of being in and knowing the world. This distinction is fundamental to the Western sense of things and ideas and sets the frame in which knowledge about the world as nature can be gathered through theories, leading to a stable representation of the world that can be carried around and worked on in the realm of empirical, context-dependent knowledge.

Initiation into "dreaming" can be sudden and results from a significant dream. In my experience, the dreaming that was important for others, in a moment became a way of dreaming for me. It was part of the Sámi knowledge tradition in the environment where I resided, and it was a form of knowing that could be recalled by an ethnographer who was struggling to learn something that was (partly) forgotten, sometimes doing homework more than fieldwork. Ingmar had become my teacher with regard to dreaming. On the night that he died, I had a dream: Ingmar is riding a bus on his way home; I am standing beside the highway when he passes by, leaving me behind. The dream woke me up; my sense was that he had come to me. In the morning his relatives called me. When I told them that I had been dreaming about him, this made perfect sense to them. For them, he had called my name. I had been dreaming Ingmar, not dreaming *about* him. This is an important distinction. The dreaming remade the connection between him and me, and he could call my name. I stayed open to guidance via a dream, one could say, and learned to take seriously the connections made, even though they are still not clearly formed but are more of a hunch. The dream provides clarity. The dreaming is therefore an entrance into connections and communities.

An ethnographic story highlights this argument. Some years after this initial dream with Ingmar I was doing ethnographic work, together with fellow researcher Kirsten Stien, on Russian prostitution in Finnmark County. This project came about because of a new situation in the North: prostitution had become a solution for some Russian women in the economic and politically challenging times after the collapse of the Soviet state and the opening of the border with Russia in 1989. Families on the Kola Peninsula suffered great disadvantages, and some people took advantage of this and organized trafficking; we, as researchers, were asked to look into the situation. We arrived late at night and stayed with Ester, a Sámi woman, who offered rooms, meals, and healing in her home; she also hosted tourists in her guesthouse. During dinner Ester introduced us to the area by telling stories about the people, places, and former political processes that she saw as being important and relevant. The atmosphere was friendly, and we reflected upon all those stories that came out of the area in relation to Russian prostitution. We knew that some years earlier a camp had been set up where Russian women and Norwegian men could meet. This drew media attention, and the public focus on this activity in the village was inescapable. Everybody had to take a stand, and a painful debate began, using the media as the channel for the mediation of the different opinions. For our study we made a plan in the form of a list of people to contact. The list comprised mostly people in formal positions, all of whom had a strong voice in the public discourse on the issue. Then we went to bed. We were sleeping in a *gamme*[2] that had been set up for housing the tourists and travellers who came to Ester's farm.

That night I had a dream. I was walking through streets in a city crowded with people. They were selling and buying, playing and laughing. There were only familiar faces—everywhere. I knew them all, but I did not stop. I was in a hurry, but I was capable of enjoying the smell of the city at the same time. Suddenly I found myself at the beginning of the tundra. There was a long, long way ahead of me, and a shapeless shape was moving. It was changing, taking up new forms as I was watching. Its creator had power over me, and I was pulled toward him or her and could not resist. All I knew was that this was evil, and if I came closer I would see his or her face. And I knew that the only solution was to fight my way out of the dream. I did. Lying awake in bed in this *gamme* in Polmak, I listened to my heart beating. I was not frightened, but shaken. Then I moved into sleep and fell directly into the same spot on the tundra; the evil was taking me in, pulling me closer to become visible before me. I knew I had to take up the same fight all over again and that the only way to resist his face was to leave the dream. And it was possible; I managed to leave in time. I woke up. I left the bed and went into the shower. The morning broke. I waited for Kirsten, my college friend, to wake up. When she did, we had breakfast, and I told her the story from my sleepless night. Our decision was clear; we took the car and drove off. Both of us knew that we had to rethink our plans and our understanding related to the project. We had come there to start the project, but we made an abrupt about-face to reconsider.

The dream had a clear message for both of us: it was necessary to leave behind what had been said in public about prostitution in this village. It was a powerful dream that reminded us to be open to differences and to try to be conscious of the moral discourse of which I was already a part, and thereby to not decide (that is, accept any one story of what the evil face looked like) before we had carried out our own ethnographic work. Instead of our original plan of talking to the governmental body of the municipality, we decided to commence by asking to participate in the everyday life of one of the houses where Norwegian men and Russian women met. The evil appearing in the dream became a reminder to not come with foregone conclusions and categories of reality, but to let the ethnographic work inform us in relation to lived realities. Our steps were the following: we entered one of the houses and stood in the hallway, explaining that we were interested in the people's point of view. We were invited in and had coffee. We stayed day and night for some weeks, doing the cooking, washing the dishes, shopping for groceries, and sitting at the kitchen table talking to people who came, and our engagement offered a normal gender appearance in a home where this was most welcome. With regard to the change we made in our research project, we can refer to several authors: a more generous sense of method appeared through the project (Markussen, 2006) that could be articulated as a reflexive, embodied engagement with otherness that foregrounds the deconstructive work offered by Spivak (1985/1994); "that which helps us think against ourselves" (Lather, 2010, p. 84); or it could be reframed as indigenous methodology (Smith, 1999).

Decolonization in Sápmi

The act of recalling the interconnectedness of people, land, the spiritual, the past, and the present is part of the ongoing decolonization in Sápmi. It is a political project on which new governmental bodies are working, and still the recollection is also about mourning the separation and disruption created throughout the assimilation period. The Sámi woman Inga, who grew up in the 1960s, explained:

> When I grew up—it was not meant to be that we girls should have a life in reindeer herding, at least not in our area. I come from a reindeer-herding family. We learned that we should find a job, marry a southerner, and just come back to our land on vacations. I'm only "half taught" at being a proper reindeer-herding woman. Even though I grew up with it, I never had the possibility to be skilled. Furthermore, I did not have the possibility to mediate this knowledge and pass it on to my children the way I would have wanted. Some things I managed, but there is still a long way to go...
>
> There are times when I think about that part of my life. It demands for me not only that I cannot find the words that I need, but what I must do is to inspect myself on a more fundamental level and excuse the woman I have become and the woman I should have been—and nobody knows about this.

Butler (2004) addresses mourning, not as mimicry but as a practice through which the past is remembered and restored. Mourning, she argues, should be seen as a way of reliving an area. When the past is brought into the present, an opportunity opens for entering into a dialogue with what was lost and what remains from losing it. In these moments, mourning becomes oddly fecund and paradoxically productive (Butler, 2004). Recalling interconnectedness through the analysis of "following the gift" addresses the process of decolonization.

While the loss of connection to knowledge traditions—and, by that, the possibility of considering oneself as skilled (the example of Inga above)—is precisely the consequence of living in colonized times, it is integral to those very colonial dynamics in which the pains that result are carried more by individuals than by what has been the case traditionally, the community. When, for example, individuals such as Inga are drawn out of the often nomadic and subsistence-oriented livelihoods and take up work in government, enrol their children in schools, or develop their farming, fishing, harvesting, or reindeer husbandry according to the national standards—in short, enter the market economy as well as the welfare state—this may bring benefits in the short term; however, it also involves experiences of disconnection that are suffered most intensely on an individual level where people may also feel overwhelmed by effects such as shame, grief, and anger. Still, what appears in my stories is that epistemic practices such as indigenous dreaming and "following the gift" are hidden but still very much alive, whereby these realities are articulated into everyday life. Dreaming does not end with the dream. As I have argued, autonomy on the one hand and community on the other hand are done in the same moment. Autonomies and the obligation to respect the autonomy of others are evident in Sámi epistemic practice. It is interesting that dreaming as part of Sámi epistemic practices is similar to that of, and is in evidence among, other circumpolar people such as the Ojibwa (Hallowell, 1960), the Chipewyan (Smith, 1998), the Inuit (Guemple, 1991), Siberia nomads (Vitebsky, 2005), and the Yukaghirs (Willerslev, 2007). We could speculate that it is especially in circumpolar communities that flexibility (responding to new options, inclusive gift distribution) is understood to be a value that ensures survival and co-operation so that the ongoing renewal of cultural forms can meet the constantly changing environment that is the Arctic.

I have argued for the notion that dreaming and other indigenous spiritual practices should be noticed and taken seriously. We should also respect that this practice is multiple. Indigenous people in the contemporary societies differ, and their notion of dreaming is not the same. Still, it is important that we move toward realizing the notions of superstition or spirituality as cultural constructs, and acknowledging that dreaming is real, at least for some. It should be noted that there is no equivalent to the English concept of superstition in the Sámi language. The concept of superstition is however expressed in Norwegian (where there is an equivalent) in the concept of *overnaturlig*, which relates to beliefs that are above the reality of nature, of the everyday; this is clearly not contained in Sámi concepts.

I follow the arguments of Willerslev (2007) and Grieves (2008) that real change will begin with an appreciation of the inherent value of indigenous philosophy, where spirituality is called upon as part of the everyday and as a way of living with the land and waters. Such philosophy is not a mental representation imposed upon the world by indigenous people, but life is lived through this epistemic practice. We need to reconsider the theoretical tools by which we attempt to enter a people's relationship with dreams, spirits, souls, and land. We should also consider that such a reconsidering is important for the well-being of the indigenous people, and may well be for both people and the planet where we are given residence, even though it is only for a short term in the history of the universe. A spiritual relationship, living on and with the land and where nature is seen as sacred, should be respected; we should feel humble before it. It is an idea to be greeted and listened to, and one that can give guidance in an ethical relationship with nature, having practices that are much needed in the age of global warming and the new industrial turn in the Arctic region.

Author's Note

I want to express my gratitude to Liv Østmo, who serves as *allaskuvlaoahpa-headdji* (college teacher) at Sámi allaskuvla, for her generous reading of and comments upon this chapter.

Notes

1. *Finnmark dagblad*, March 6, 2003.
2. *A gamme* is the traditional Sámi turf hut, used as a dwelling place.

References

Alver, B.G. (1997). På hjul efter det rullende menneske Magi og det magiske som udtryk for identitet og selvforståelse. In T. Selberg (Ed.), *Utopi og besvergelse Magi i moderne kultur*, KULTS skriftserie nr. 83 (pp. 108–123). Oslo: Research Council of Norway.

Bjørklund, I., & Eidheim, H. (1999). Om reinmerker—kulturelle sammenhenger og norsk jus i Sápmi. In I. Bjørklund (Ed.), *Norsk ressursforvaltning og samiske rettighetsforhold* (pp. 143–158). Oslo: Ad Notam Gyldendal.

Butler, J. (2003). Afterword: After loss, what then? In D. Eng & D. Kazanjian (Eds.), *Loss: The politics of mourning* (pp. 467–475). Berkeley: University of California Press.

Butler, J. (2004). *Undoing gender*. New York: Routledge.

Crapanzano, V. (2003). *Imaginative horizons: An essay in literary-philosophical anthropology.* Chicago: University of Chicago Press.

Freud, S., & Oppenheim, D.E. (1958). *Dreams in folklore.* New York: International Universities Press.

Gaski, H. (2008). Nils-Aslak Valkeapää: Indigenous voice and multimedia artist. *AlterNative, an International Journal of Indigenous Peoples, 4*(2), 155–178.

Grieves, V. (2008). Aboriginal spirituality: A baseline for indigenous knowledges development in Australia. *Canadian Journal of Native Studies, 28* (2), 363–398.

Guemple, L. (1991). Teaching social relations to Inuit children. In T. Ingold, D. Riches, & J. Woodburn (Eds.), *Hunters and gatherers, II: Property, power, and ideology* (pp. 131–149). Oxford: Berg Publishers.

Hallowell, A.I. (1960). Ojibwa ontology, behaviour, and world-view. In S. Dimond (Ed.), *Culture in history: Essays in honour of Paul Radin* (pp. 19–52). New York: Columbia University Press.

Hoem, I. (1999). Representasjoner av relasjoner og forskjeller. *Norsk Antropologisk tidskrift, 10*(2), 125–149.

Kapferer, B. (1997). *The feast of the sorcerer practices of consciousness and power.* Chicago: University of Chicago Press.

Kramvig, B. (2003). Nature, culture, dreams and healing. In I.K. Pedersen & A. Viken (Eds.), *Nature and identity: Essays on the culture of nature* (pp. 167–187). Kristiansand, Norway: Høgskoleforlaget, Norwegian Academic Press.

Kramvig, B. (2005). The silent language of ethnicity. *European Journal for Cultural Studies, 8*(1), 45–64.

Kramvig, B. (2006). *Finnmarksbilder.* Doctoral thesis, University of Tromsø.

Kramvig, B. (2009). Le langage silencieux du don dans les communautés arctiques. *Ethnologie Francaise, 39*(2), 275–284.

Kuokkanen, R. (2006). The logic of the gift: Reclaiming indigenous peoples' philosophies. In T. Botz-Bornstein (Ed.), *Re-ethnicizing the mind? Cultural revival in contemporary thought* (pp. 251–257). Amsterdam and New York: Rodopi.

Kuokkanen, R. (2007). *Reshaping the university: Responsibility, indigenous episteme, and the logic of the gift.* Vancouver: University of British Columbia Press.

Kuokkanen, R. (2010). The responsibility of the academy: A call for doing homework. *Journal of Curriculum Theorizing, 26*(3), 61–74.

Lather, P. (2010). *Engaging science policy: From the side of the mess.* New York: Peter Lang.

Law, J., & Lin, W. (2011). Cultivating disconcertment. *Sociological Review, 58*(s2), 135–153.

Markussen, T. (2006). Moving worlds: The performativity of affective engagement. *Feminist Theory 7*(3), 291–308.

Mauss, M. (1990). *The gift: The form and reason for exchange in archaic societies.* London: Routledge.

Miller, B. (2007). *Connecting and correcting: A case study of Sami healers in Porsanger.* Leiden, Netherlands: CNWS.

Minde, H. (Ed.). (2008). *Indigenous peoples: Self-determination, knowledge, indigeneity.* Delft: Eburon.

Myrvoll, M. (2010). *"Bare gudsordet duger": Om kontinuitet og brudd I samiske virkelighetsforståelse.* Tromsø: Tromsø Universitetet I Tromsø, Institutt for arkeologi og sosialantropologi.

Odner, K. (1995). Samisk identitet. *Norsk Antropologisk tidskrift,* 2, 127–135.

Pehrson, R. (1964). *The bilateral network of social relations in Könkämä Lapp district.* Oslo: Universitetsforlaget.

Ricoeur, P. (2005). *The course of recognition.* Trans. D. Pellauer. London: Harvard University Press.

Sandberg, A. (2009). Constituting a new order in the European north. In F. Sabetti, B. Allen, & M. Sproule-Jones (Eds.), *The practice of constitutional development: Vincent Ostrom's quest to understand human affairs* (pp. 227–245). Lanham, MD: Lexington Books.

Sara, M.N. (2009). Siida and traditional Sami reindeer herding knowledge. *Northern Review,* 30, 153–179.

Smith, D.M. (1998). An Athapaskan way of knowing: Chipewan ontology. *American Ethnologist,* 25(3), 412–432.

Smith, L.T. (1999). *Decolonizing methodologies: Research and indigenous peoples.* London: Zed Books.

Spivak, G.C. (1985/1994). Can the subaltern speak? In P. Willians & L. Chrisman (Eds.), *Colonial discourse and post-colonial theory* (pp. 66–112). New York: Columbia University Press.

Stoller, P. (1995). *Embodying colonial memories: Spirit possession, power, and the Hauka in West Africa.* New York: Routledge.

Taussig, M. (1993). *Mimesis and alterity: A particular history of the senses.* New York: Routledge.

Verran, H. (2002). A postcolonial moment in science studies: Alternative firing regimes of environmental sciences and aboriginal landowners. *Social Studies of Science,* 32(5–6), 729–762.

Verran, H. (2004). A story about doing "the dreaming." *Postcolonial Studies,* 7(2), 149–164.

Vitebsky, P. (2005). *Reindeer people living with animals and spirits in Siberia.* London: Harpers Perennial.

Watson-Verran, H., & Turnbull, D. (1995). Science and other indigenous knowledge systems. In S. Jasanoff, G.E. Markle, J.C. Petersen, & T. Pinch (Eds.), *Handbook of science and technology studies* (pp. 115–140). London: Sage.

Willerslev, R. (2007). *Soul hunters: Hunting, animism, and personhood among the Siberian Yukaghirs.* Berkeley: University of California Press.

Contributors

KJELL BIRKELY ANDERSEN, currently working in Acute Services at Sámi National Centre for Mental Health, is a psychotherapist. He holds a master's degree in Mental Health Care. Andersen's essay, "To Recover: A Case Study of Experiences in the Coastal Sámi area," appeared in A. Silviken and V. Stordag (Eds.), *Nye Landskap kjente steder og skjulte utfordringer* (Karasjok, Norway: ČálliidLágádus, 2010).

ANNE KAREN HÆTTA completed her master's degree in Indigenous Studies at the University of Tromsø in 2010. Previously she had been working in research projects on health, livelihoods, migration, and identity at the Centre for Sámi Health Research at the University of Tromsø. She is currently working in the Árbediehtu project at Sámi University College, which aims to collect, document, and systematize the Sámi traditional knowledge related to the understanding and the use of nature.

MONA ANITA KIIL is a Research Fellow in the Department of Clinical Medicine, Faculty of Health Sciences at UiT The Arctic University of Norway. She has a master's degree in Social Anthropology and is currently studying for her doctorate in Medical Anthropology; her thesis will examine cultural perspectives on mental health in Northern Norway. Kiil's research interests are broad and include identity processes and dynamics of belonging, post-colonialism, ethnicity and indigenous people, modernity, religion, ritual, gender, mental health, traditional medicine, alternative and complementary medicine, food, and body and embodiment. Kiil has done fieldwork in West Africa and Northern Norway.

BRITT KRAMVIG, PhD, is a professor in the Department of Tourism and Northern Studies, UiT The Arctic University of Norway. Her ethnographic work has taken place in the Arctic and within the field of post-colonial, indigenous, and cultural studies. Kramvig takes inspiration from feminist theory and science and technology studies, as well as phenomenology. Her recent publications are part of the ongoing research project "Arctic Encounters, Traveling and Travel Writing in the European High North," financed by Humanities in the European Research Area (HERA), as well as the research project "Reason to Return," financed by the Norwegian Research Council.

TRINE KVITBERG is a doctoral candidate in Health Science at the Department of Community Medicine, the Arctic University of Norway. She holds a master's degree in Social Anthropology, a master's degree in Public Health, and a bachelor's degree in Nursing. Her research interests include medical anthropology, health, culture, food, human rights, personal biographies, visual cultural studies, and anthropology of the senses.

STEIN R. MATHISEN, PhD, Folklore Studies, is a professor of Culture Studies at the Arctic University of Norway, Finnmark Faculty Alta, where he teaches heritage tourism in the master's program of Tourist Studies. Major research interests include folk medicine and folk belief, the role of narratives in the constitution of identity and ethnicity, questions of heritage politics and ethno-politics, and the history of cultural research in the northern areas. He has conducted fieldwork in various Kven, Sámi, and Norwegian locations in Northern Norway concerning identity, ethnicity, folk medicine, and folk belief, and in the Finn Forest area (Norway and Sweden) concerning festivals and revitalization of ethnic culture.

Recently published articles in English include "Narrated Sámi Sieidis: Heritage and Ownership in Ambiguous Border Zones," *Ethnologia Europaea*, 39(2), 2009, 11–25; and "Indigenous Spirituality in the Touristic Borderzone: Virtual Performances of Sámi Shamanism in Sápmi Park," *Temenos*, 46(1), 2010, 53–72.

BARBARA HELEN MILLER, PhD in Anthropology from Leiden University in the Netherlands, is currently an independent scholar, working in co-operation with Research Group Circumpolar Cultures. She received a master's degree in the Psychology of Religion from Norwich University, Vermont College, in the United States and a diploma in Analytical Psychology from the C.G. Jung Institute Zürich in Switzerland. Her most widely read publication is *Connecting and Correcting: A Case Study of Sámi Healers in Porsanger* (Leiden: CNWS, 2007).

MARIT MYRVOLL, PhD, is a social anthropologist and museum manager at Várdobáiki Sámi Museum in Norway. She is interested primarily in the field of cultural heritage, and her research focus has for long been continuity and change in the Sámi religious world view. The range of her research experience includes working with Tibetans in exile, the Maronite minority in Cyprus, and the Sámi people in Norway, Sweden, and Finland. She has been working in the Sámi parliament in Norway and also in national and regional cultural heritage management. Her concerns include Sámi educational issues on all levels, from elementary school to university. As a Sámi politician, Myrvoll has for several decades been engaged in the development and strengthening of Sámi higher education and its research. Her current research area is the High North, focusing on challenges concerning the indigenous (Sámi) as well as other minorities and national cultural heritage, which ranges from local intangible cultural heritage to the UNESCO world heritage sites in Norway and the Nordic countries.

RANDI NYMO, a registered nurse with a doctorate in Health Science, is an associate professor at Narvik University College. She is a specialist in both psychiatrics and intensive care, as well as an authorized supervisor. As a young Sámi from Northern Norway, she developed an ethno-political commitment. During her professional career she has engaged extensively in the care of Sámi patients. Her main interest is cultural nursing with focus on practices developed by the Sámi to cope with everyday challenges, health, and disease management. Nymo continues to explore understandings of health, illness, and rehabilitation. Sámi experiences with cultural and political suppression have influenced Sámi identity management and language use. Nymo is very devoted to these conditions in her research.

SIGVALD PERSEN, a civil engineer, was employed by Porsanger Municipality for some 30 years. For the last 10 years he has been the manager of the Sámi Cultural Centre (Mearrasámi diehtoguovddáš) in Porsanger. His website, www.meron.no, is often consulted for research.

Index

Geertz, Clifford, 52, 99
Giddens, A., 63–64
gift giving, 195–196, 197–198, 198–199
gifts of grace, 60, 61–62, 66
Goffman, E., 162, 164, 167, 168, 172, 174
Grieves, V., 204
gufihttarat (subterraneous beings), 74–75, 80
gurus, and knowledge, 36
guvhllár (traditional healer), 28. *See also* Sámi
    traditional healers

Hanem, Torild, 30
Hansen, John, 177–178
Harrison, S., 40
healers, *see* Sámi traditional healers
health, 51–53. *See also* Sámi traditional healing
health-care systems
    Kleinman's model, 51–52, 54, 137, 162, 174
hermeneutic phenomenology, 164
Hildegard, collaborative ethnography of
    approach to, 83–84
    aggressive stance of Hildegard, 96
    gane in, 93–94, 97
    health narrative of, 89–94
    modern medicine in, 84, 98
    participation in, 95–96, 98–99, 101
    transcultural psychiatry in, 100–101
    Western *vs.* traditional diagnoses, 101
Hobsbawm, E., 151
Hoem, I., 197–198
home, 142, 150–151
Hultkrantz, Å, 81n2

identity, *see* Sámi identity
idioms of health and healing, *see* multiple
    discourses, engagement with
illness, conceptions of, 54–55, 57
illness narratives, 126
Imaginative Horizons (Crapanzano), 191
indigenous episteme, 186–187, 194
indigenous knowledge, 3–4, 20, 160–161, 186.
    See also traditional knowledge
indigenous philosophy, 160–161, 204
indigenous researchers, 164
inspirational healing, xxi, xxii
Intergovernmental Panel on Climate Change
    (IPCC), 104, 128n2

internat (boarding school) experience, 89, 96
International Women's Day, 128n8

Jernsletten, J., 127
Johansen, R.E., 39
juovssaheaddji (one who returns), 76. *See also*
    Sámi traditional healers

Kaaven, Johan, 16, 76–77, 80–81
Kalstad, J.K.H., 158
Kapferer, B., 189–190
Karasjok, Norway, 152n1
Kassam, K.-A. S., 122–123
Kateb, G., 151
kinship, *see* Sámi kinship systems
Kirmayer, Laurence, 99
Kleinman, Arthur
    cultural formulation and, 99
    health-care systems and, 51–52, 54, 137, 162,
        174
    on illness *vs.* disease, 64
knowledge, *see* indigenous philosophy; secrecy,
    in traditional healing knowledge
knowledge management, 36, 40–41
Kohl-Larsen, Ludwig, 13
Kola Peninsula, 105. *See also* women, elderly
    Russian Sámi
Kola Sámi creation myth, 122–123
Komi people, 105–106, 128n4
Körningk, Johan F., 5–6
Kull lumm (fish soup), 128n7, 133
Kuokkanen, Rauna, 186–187, 196, 198–199
Kuutma, Kristin
    Collaborative Representations, 14
Kven people, 134, 135

læsinga (readings), 43n1
Laestadian First Born Congregation, Måsske,
    48, 49, 67n3
Laestadianism
    ethnic inclusiveness of, xxvn1, 136–137
    on good and bad spiritual connection, 96,
        97
    on "good thoughts," 85
    in Hildegard's life, 93
    in Johanna's life, 146
    on neo-shamanism, 65

Moe, Jørgen, 12
Moe, Moltke, 12
Montin, Lars, 8
Moroccan mystical thinking, 191
mourning, 194, 203
Muittalus samid birra (Turi), 14–16, 53–54
multiple discourses, engagement with
    in Andersen's work, 85–87, 88–89
    approach to, 83–84
    transcultural psychiatry, 100–101
Myandash creation myth, 122
Myrvoll, Marit, 26, 28

Nakata, M., 164
naming
    approach to, xxiii, 73, 81
    baptism and, 74–75, 75–76, 77–78, 80
    competition story, 75–76, 81
    as correction, 75, 77–78
    dynamics of, 72–73
    fishing boat story, 73–74
    as forceful and determining, 76–77
    grandchild story, 74–75
    local expressions of, 71–72
    as names having meanings, 73–74, 78–79
    neighbour's daughter (Kaaven) story,
        76–77, 81
    Pentikäinen on, 79–80
    renaming, 78, 80, 81
    returning of "bad" and, 81
    rude man story, 77–78, 81
    spiritual connection of names, 81
Nanna (Persen's mother), 95, 96
nature, 85, 178. See also *ulda* (little people)
neavrrit (evils), 30
neo-shamanism, xxii, 28, 65, 66
Nergård, Jens-Ivar, 72
nested dialogues, 141
neuroscience, 99
noaidi/noajdde
    appointment of, 62
    Christianity and, 33, 58
    definition of, 43n3
    Laestadianism and, 96
    Myrvoll on, 28
    role and status of, 56–57
    use of term, 21n1, 67n8

See also Sámi traditional healers
Noble Savage myth, 3, 7
Nordreisa, Norway, 134, 135, 139, 144
northern Troms, 132, 134–135
northern Troms mental health study
    home and clinic as different cultural arenas,
        149–150, 151–152
    home and unhomely, 142, 150–151
    intersection between traditional and
        conventional healing, 146–149
    Johanna's story, 143–148, 151
    methodology and ethics, 138–141
    Thor on identity, 131
Norway
    folklore studies in, 11–12
    health services in, 133
    Sámi in, xx
    treatment of minorities in, 134
Norwegianization
    decolonization of, 185–186
    in education, 9–10, 170–171
    history of, 158–159, 179n2
    impact on agriculture, 174–175
    impact on traditional healing, 34, 50, 57
    in Markebygd region, 157–158, 161, 178
    Sámi cultural renaissance and, 167–168

Odner, Knut, 189
openness, degrees of, 26
Oppenheim, D.E., 193
ordinary life, 107–108
Oskal, Nils, 127
Overing, J., 142, 150

pain, 55, 121–122, 129n9
Paine, Robert, 72
participation, 95–96, 98–99, 101
Pehrson, R., 196, 197
Pentikäinen, J., 79–80
perogies, 128n8
Persen, Sigvald, 94–96, 97
pietism, xxi–xxii, 48
political autonomy, 187
Pollan, B., 57
pollution, 103–104, 105. *See also* women, elderly
    Russian Sámi
Porsanger, Norway, xxiii–xxiv. *See also* naming

Sámi health issues, research on, 132–134
Sámi identity
    breakdown of in Russia, 107
    complexity of, 131, 134–135, 139, 183–184
    health and, 131–132, 133
    hiding of, 166
    idioms of health and, 83
    Laestadianism and, 136–137
    See also home; Norwegianization
Sámi idioms of health and healing, see multiple
        discourses, engagement with
Sámi kinship systems, 162, 196, 197–198
Sámi language, xix–xx, 159, 170, 183
Sámi spirituality
    Christianization of, xxi–xxii, 48–49, 179n2
    cultural identity and, 183–184
    health and healing and, 56
    nature and, 127, 160
    overview of, xx–xxi
    persecution of, 33–34, 57–58, 158–159, 160
    reconsidering, 204–205
    reindeer in, 122
    See also Laestadianism; Sámi dreaming
        epistemology
Sámi traditional healers
    abilities of, 60
    categories of, 28
    charismatic authority of, 38, 66
    consulting, and cultural values, 65–66
    contemporary, xxi
    embedded context of, 55
    healers on being, 62–63, 94–96
    as inspirational, xxi, xxii
    legitimacy of, 35–36, 66–67
    loss of abilities, 61
    low profile kept by, 32–33, 94
    pre-Christian, xxi
    qualifications for, 31–32
    reasons for being interviewed, 35–36
    source of abilities, 60–61
    specialization among, 29, 59–60
    terms for, 28, 49, 67n4, 76–77
    transmission of knowledge, xxii–xxiii,
        30–31, 60–61, 62, 66
    Western medicine and, 49–50
    See also secrecy, in traditional healing
        knowledge

Sámi traditional healing
    alternative medicine and, 42–43
    caution in, 96
    changing norms for, 42
    Christianity and, 56, 57, 61–63, 66
    contemporary, 58–59, 63
    criminalization of, 34, 50, 57
    historical practice of, 56–58
    Laestadianism and, xxii, 96, 135–137
    mental illness in, 30
    neo-shamanism and, 65
    origins of, 27–28, 53
    overview of methods, 29
    pain and, 55
    participation as element of, 95–96, 99
    relationship in between users and
        practitioners, 47, 58–59, 63–64, 65–66
    results from Andersen's research on, 85
    for social relationships, 101, 158
    Western medicine and, 53–54, 63, 64, 87,
        88–89, 92–93, 98, 172–174
    See also cupping; naming; reading;
        Sámi traditional healers; secrecy, in
        traditional healing knowledge
Sámi traditional knowledge, 26. See also
        indigenous knowledge; traditional
        authority
Sandberg, Georg, 12
SANKS (Sámi Competence Centre for
        Psychiatric Health Care), 84–85
scholarly research, see Sámi folk medicine, in
        scholarly research initiatives
school medicine, see Western medicine
Sea Sámi, see Coastal Sámi
secrecy, in traditional healing knowledge
    introduction to, 26–27
    borders between secret and open
        knowledge, 41–42, 55–56
    continued relevance of, 42
    maintenance of, 38–39, 39–40
    in practice, 56, 60, 66–67
    preservation and, 26–27
    qualifications for guvhllár and, 32
    reasons for, 36–37
    stories illustrating, 25–26, 39–40
secret knowledge, 26
sensitive listening, 108–109

Other Titles from The University of Alberta Press

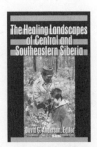

THE HEALING LANDSCAPES OF CENTRAL
AND SOUTHEASTERN SIBERIA
David G. Anderson, Editor
Patterns of Northern Traditional Healing Series
194 pages | 48 photographs, references, glossary, index
978-1-896445-58-8 | $40.00 (T) paper
Traditional Medicine | Siberia | Russia

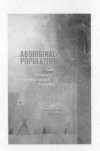

ABORIGINAL POPULATIONS
Social, Demographic, and Epidemiological Perspectives
Frank Trovato and Anatole Romaniuk, Editors
600 pages | Tables, figures, map, notes, bibliography, index
978-0-88864-625-5 | $60.00 (T) paper
978-1-77212-032-5 | $47.99 (T) PDF
Native Studies | Sociology | Demography

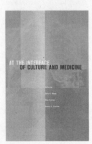

AT THE INTERFACE OF CULTURE AND MEDICINE
Earle H. Waugh, Olga Szafran & Rodney A. Crutcher, Editors
316 pages | Maps, figures, bibliography, index
978-0-88864-532-6 | $49.95 (T) paper
978-0-88864-639-2 | $39.99 (T) PDF
Medicine | Cultural Studies